THE SECOND HALF
BEGINS
AT 50...

YOUR LONGEVITY
HANDBOOK

BABY BOOMER SERIES
PUBLICATION

BY
OTHNIEL J. SEIDEN, MD&
JANE L. BILETT, PhD, CLINICAL PSYCHOLOGIST

Cover Art
by Capri Brock

Proudly Published in the USA by
Thornton Publishing, Inc
17011 Lincoln Ave. #408
Parker, CO 80134

Phone: 303.794.8888
Fax: 720.863.2013

BooksToBelieveIn.com/Health.php

BoomerBookSeries.com

ISBN: 1519496389

For Our children &
grandchildren

May they live to 120
healthy, happy years!

TABLE OF CONTENTS

Chapter 1

May You Live to Be 120...

Virtually all recent medical research on aging points to the fact that the human animal, you and me included, has the potential to live up to 120 years of age.

That means you and I can live 120 active, happy and productive years—not years in a rocking chair, wheel chair or nursing home. That being the case, THE SECOND HALF of our lives does indeed BEGIN AT 50.... However, since most of us have spent the first part of our lives mistreating our God given equipment, this human body of ours; so we may not all make it to 120. But the good news is that most of us should be able to make it to 100 and well over.

This book is dedicated at giving us the best possible chance at reaching as near as possible to our true life potential.

Let's re-emphasize, **we are talking about healthy, happy, active and productive years full of the things we enjoy doing.** We are talking about adding years to our lives—and more important—putting **quality life in our remaining years.**

How often have you heard the question, "If you had it to do over again, what would you change?" Well, if you are coming up on 50, theoretically, you do have it all to do over again. Just think what you should be able to do with those years, knowing all that you've learned in the first 50! What you need to do is get yourself into the best shape you can, so you can live out as much of your 120 year potential as possible. It is to that end, that this book is committed. Follow this program, and within a year you should be as fit as you can be, and headed for as bright and long a future as possible, **may you live to 120!**

Still a little skeptical about all those studies that say we should be full of fun, vigor and productive activity to 120 years of age? Just look around at what's going on in the rest of this world, and not too far from home, I might add. It might surprise you to know just how many people over 100 years of age are living right here in the United States; would you believe over 100,000? That's 50,000 more than just ten years ago and that number is expected to pass 125,000 in just a few years. We've learned a lot about aging in the past decade. But this kind of longevity is not new. In other parts of the world, people have been living remarkably long life spans.

I work as medical director to an organization, **Doctors To The World,** which sends volunteer medical personnel into 'areas of need' the world over. This gives me the opportunity to go to some fascinating places, most of them in the Third World. It was a surprise to me that health in the Third World is often better than here in America.

We've all heard of the starvation and terrible diseases in places like India, Bangladesh, Somalia, in the Sudan, but these are really exceptions rather than the rule. These situations make the news, as well they should, to arouse our interest to give aid. Less frequently do we hear about the Third World people who live nine to ten decades or longer—we mean active and productive decades.

One of my first exposures to these long living Third World people was in one of the most primitive places on earth, Zone Makita, Honduras. Life in this area goes on pretty much as it has, unchanged, for over six-hundred years. The area has few roads, virtually no electricity or other modern technology. I was among people who had never seen a modern doctor, having been cared for only "Medicine Chiefs" when they were ill. Herbs, teas and potions were the main medicinals of the area. Their elderly were active into their late nineties and there were more than just a few of them.

Barbuda is a small island in the Caribbean, just twenty-eight miles due north of Antigua. It has only about 1200 residents, all living in one small village at the edge of a large lagoon. There only medical care is provided mainly by volunteer doctors who rotate to the island a month at a time. But even before we provided them with volunteer medical care, these people were living into their nineties and past one-hundred—and as in Honduras, they remain active and productive.

In Ecuador, I was introduced to real longevity. I was with a team of Ophthalmologists and nurses, volunteers who replaced three-hundred cataracts with intra-ocular lenses. My job was to examine all the patients to make sure they were able to withstand surgery. I also examined numerous others who were there for other eye treatments. Altogether I checked over five-hundred of the natives of that area of Ecuador, high in the Andes mountains, at an altitude of about 10,000 feet. Among those five-hundred people I found no heart disease, no cancer, no diabetes, no evidence of stroke or hypertension—all the diseases that kill off Americans in our fifth, sixth and seventh decades of life. Granted, the people who had these dreaded diseases may not have come in for eye problems, but I doubt that. In any case, I was examining natives in their 30s, 40s, 50s, 60s, 70s, 80s, 90s, people 100, 102, 106, one as old as 114. And these people were leading active lives, most having walked several miles to come to our hospital in the town of Granada. Furthermore, I was told, we were not too far from a village where people lived over 100 routinely—one reportedly over 130 years.

Armenia is a country deprived of our high tech medical

system and her people suffer severe economic hardships. I was privileged to lead one of two American medical teams into that country immediately after her devastating earthquake of 1988. In the major city of Yeravan, life expectancy did not seem any different than ours; lower in fact on the average. There men died in mid to late fifties and women in their later sixties. These city people were exposed to pollution and stress equal to any of our major cities. They smoked and ate a high fat diet even beyond our levels of indulgence. The only place their habits improved on those of Americans was that they were a bit less sedentary than we. But outside of their capitol city it was quite another story. In the mountain villages where the diet was considerably healthier, the air far cleaner, the lifestyle more relaxed and tobacco use virtually unknown, where the people walked several miles a day to get from one place to another, those people lived long active lives. Late 90s` 100 to 110 years of longevity are not uncommon; 120 to 130 are less common but not unheard of, and the world's oldest recorded age of 147 came from that area.

The point is, that we Americans are only living 1/2 to 2/3 of our allotted time on this earth and we aren't fit enough to fully enjoy the years that we do survive. The good news is that we can do something about it if we want and the changes we have to make in our life style aren't that drastic or painful.

In spite of the fact that, in the past decades American's life spans have lengthened dramatically.

There is plenty of room for our improvement!

This book will lead you through those changes. Make them and you'll be amazed at how much health, activity, fun, productivity and ambition can be returned to your old bones. Your goal, **"should you accept this assignment,"** is to become as fit as you can possibly be by this time next year, heading for a bright and long happy, healthy, active and productive future.

CHAPTER 2

WORKING TOWARD YOUR MAXIMUM POTENTIAL....

> American's longevity is only
> forty-second in the world,
> and many of those countries
> ahead of us are
> Third World countries!

The human animal was designed to live to about 120 years of age, there's little doubt about that fact. And there's little doubt that the main reasons we don't achieve that age in good health is that we sabotage our own well being by the way we pollute our environs, poison our bodies, mistreat and misuse ourselves, malnourish our systems and create problems that tend to worry us to death.

A lot of you who are reading this book will ask, probably tongue-in-cheek, "Who wants to live past ninety?"

The answer to that is simple, "Almost anyone who is just turned 89!"

The truth is, most of us, the vast majority of us, want to live as long as possible if our longevity can be quality time filled with energy and good health. That's our aim. To achieve this goal, we will seek to alter our lifestyles to emulate those of the people who are already accomplishing ten or more decades of active, fulfilling, happy life. When we examine these lifestyles, there are four aspects that are common to all of them; nutrition, exercise, lack of exposure to environmental poisons and minimal distress. These peoples have been living their healthy lifestyle for centuries, a lifestyle that our scientists in the last decade have determined to be ideal for good health and long life. It's not that their ancestors were so much smarter than the rest of the world population; it's just that fate dealt them a good hand by making their environment and conditions dictate healthy habits for them.

Fortunately the changes in your lifestyle necessary to emulate them will not be as drastic as you suspect. Also we will try to just change one habit system at a time, so as not to overwhelm. The following chapters will guide you to your healthier, more active and productive long life.

LONGEVITY AND LIFESPAN STATISTICS

World wide life expectancy from birth, has risen from 46 years in 1950-1955 to 65 years in 2000-2005 and is expected to keep on rising to reach 75 years by 2045-2050. In the more developed regions, the projected increase is from 75 years today to 82 years by mid-century. Among the least developed countries, where life expectancy today is just under 50 years, it is expected to be 66 years in 2045-2050. In the rest of the developing world, under similar conditions, life expectancy is projected to rise from just under 66 years today to 76 years by mid-century.

There are close to 36 million people aged 65 and older in the United States. By the year 2050, that number is projected to rise to 87 million. The National Center for Health Statistics, dated October 10, 2001, American males born in 2000 now enjoy an average life expectancy of 74.1 years. Females born in the same year have an average life expectancy of 79.5 years. Though women can still expect to live longer than men on the average, the gap continues a narrowing trend. The 7-year difference between the sexes in life expectancy in1990 has dropped to 5.5 years.

In spite of the fact that only about 1 in 10,000 people in developed countries live to be a hundred or more, these centenarians are among one fastest-growing age groups in the United States. The U.S. Census Bureau estimates that there were between 69,000 and 81,000 centenarians living in the United States in 2000. In France, Japan and Switzerland, men and women aged 65 now live several years longer than they do in the United States. Asian-American women living in Bergen County, N.J., lead the nation in longevity, frequently reaching 91 years and older. Lowest longevity is among American Indian men in parts of South Dakota, who die around age 58. Whites in Appalachia and the Mississippi Valley die four years sooner than other Americans. Asian-Americans have a life expectancy of 84.9 years.

Regional life expectancies differ significantly. Northern residents have a life expectancy of 79 years. Middle Americans have a life expectancy of 77.9 years. Low income whites in Appalachia, Mississippi Valley have a life expectancy of only 75 years.

Western American Indians can have a life expectancy of 72.7 years. Black Middle Americans have a life expectancy of 72.9 years. Southern low-income rural blacks have a life expectancy of 71.2 years and high-risk urban blacks have a life expectancy of 71.1 years.

In Okinawa, Japan the Ministry of Health, Labor, and Welfare put out a list of average life spans by municipality for fiscal year 2000. Tomigusuku City ranked number one in Japan for women, 89.2 years and for men, the leading average lifespan of 80.6 years was held by Wara Village of Gifu Prefecture.

Life expectancy by states varies considerably too. Hawaii

has the nation's longest life expectancy at 80 years

**Other state life expectancies are in alphabetical order;
Ala. 74.4 48, Alaska 77.1 26, Ariz. 77.5 22, Ark. 75.2 43,
Calif. 78.2 10, Colo. 78.2 12, Conn. 78.7 4, Del. 76.8 29,
D.C. 72 51, Fla. 77.5 21, Ga. 75.3 41, Hawaii 80.0, Idaho
77.9 15, Ill. 76.4 33, Ind. 76.1 37, Iowa 78.3 7, Kan. 77.3 24,
Ky. 75.2 42, La. 74.2 49, Maine 77.6 20, Md. 76.3 35, Mass.
78.4 5, Mich. 76.3 34, Minn. 78.8 2, Miss. 73.6 50, Mo. 75.9
38, Mont. 77.2 25, Neb. 77.8 16, Nev. 75.8 39, N.H. 78.3 6,
N.J. 77.5 23, N.M. 77.0 27, N.Y. 77.7 19, N.C. 75.8 40, N.D.
78.3 8, Ohio 76.2 36, Okla. 75.2 44, Ore. 77.8 17, Pa. 76.7
31, R.I. 78.3 9, S.C. 74.8 47, S.D. 77.7 18, Tenn. 75.1 45,
Texas 76.7 30, Utah 78.7 3, Vt. 78.2 11,Va. 76.8 28,Wash.
78.2 13, W.Va. 75.1 46**

Life expectancy in the United States is at all an all-time high, according the United Sates Census Bureau reporting that Americans currently live an average of 77.6 years. Women live slightly longer than men do, but even more impressive is that people living to be at least 100 years old are the fastest growing segment of the population! About 80 percent of centenarians are women.

Just a few generations ago, in our lifetime memories, men in their late forties were considered old. Now, we are commonly living to be more than two times that age; in fact, living full, active and productive lives.

The older U.S. population is growing rapidly as baby boomers age; in fact, the first baby boomers will turn 65 in 2011. People age 65 and over will probably represent 20 percent of the total U.S. population by 2030, as compared to 12 percent in 2003. Yet, the Americans are youngsters compared to other developed countries, having a lower proportion of adults age 65 and older than most countries in Western Europe.

Death rates from heart disease are declining among people 65 years and older; though it still continues to be the leading cause of death within this population, followed by cancer and stroke. The rates of disability and functional limitation among the older population have declined substantially over the past two decades; about 1-in-5 older Americans report having chronic disability. This is partly due to healthier life styles, environmental education and laws and restorative surgeries and treatments. However, data comparing Americans ages 65 to 74 in 1988-94 to 1999-2000 show a startling rise in the percentage of people considered obese; for men, the proportion grew from about 24 to 33 percent and for women the figures changed (no pun intended) from about 27 percent to 39 percent.

There is a distinct possibility that if our children and grand children don't change their eating and exercise habits, they may be the first generations that live shorter life spans than their parents and grandparents!

Three-out-of-4 older people lived in metropolitan areas in 2000. There is a strong correlation between education and health. Older adults are becoming more educated, and this continuing trend could have a positive effect on the health of older people in the future: Estimates indicate that by 2030 more than one-fourth of the older population will have at least a bachelor's degree; and the percentage of older women with a bachelor's degree will likely double. The gender gap in college education will narrow in the future as younger men and women are entering and earning college degrees at roughly the same rate.

As employed men and women age, the likelihood of their working part time increases. In 2003, about half of employed men age 70 and over and almost two-thirds of employed women aged 70 and over worked part time. So far Social

Security continues to provide the largest share of income for many older Americans.

Three-quarters of the millions older Americans living alone today are women, the proportion growing greatly by age. In 2000, 4.5 percent of people ages 75 to 84 and 18.2 percent of those 85 and older lived in nursing homes. About 75% of nursing-home residents are women.

Source: U.S. Census Bureau; The report; 65+ in the United States: 2005

CHAPTER 3

GET BACK INTO SHAPE

Getting back into shape implies that you were once in good shape. If you weren't as fit as you should have been in the past, it should make little difference to our longevity goals now. This exercise program should work for you as well. It is based on the exercise that is most prevalent among the people who are outliving us by three to five decades. In recent years, it has been discovered by our exercise physiologists and sports medicine physicians to be the most beneficial and safe aerobic exercise that man and womankind can participate in. Because of the primitive conditions in the areas where our long lived counterparts live, they walk from four to twelve miles a day— and low-and-behold, walking is the best exercise to develop a strong and healthy cardiovascular system and to keep our muscles and joints functioning into our golden decades. No, you won't have to walk twelve miles a day, but a brisk walk for 45 minutes to an hour a day will make your worn out carcass over into a stronger healthier functioning body.

Let's take a look at what a daily brisk walk will do for you:

WHY A WALKING PROGRAM?

It's aerobic. It will help reduce your body fat. It will condition your heart, lungs and body. It will help lower your cholesterol and blood pressure. Walking will add years to your life and life to your years!

Walking is the most natural, safest, most perfect aerobic exercise for the human animal to participate in!

The simple secret to weight and body fat control is:

If you ingest more calories than you burn, you'll store excess body fat and your fat to lean body mass ratio will increase.

If you burn off more calories than you ingest you'll gradually burn off that storage fat to make up the needed energy and your body fat to lean body mass will decrease.

Thus, if you can increase your exercise during the day, you will also increase the amount of body fat you burn off. In addition, the exercise should tone and build muscle which increases your lean body mass. And since muscle mass burns many more calories than fat, even while at rest, your metabolic rate will increase causing your body to utilize far more calories at rest or exercise. Muscles burn 38 times more calories than fat even at rest, greatly increasing your body metabolism. This will favorably alter your body fat ratio and move you toward your ideal body weight. This does not necessarily mean you'll lose weight. Remember, fat is lighter than lean body tissue and you may actually gain weight in the exchange, but it will be an exchange of healthy muscle tissue for fat. Not a bad deal!

So what is the next step?

FIRST, TALK IT OVER WITH YOUR DOCTOR!

If you are recovering from a heart problem, of course your cardiologist must be made aware of any activity you hope to undertake. If you are a spouse, friend or relative of a heart patient and want to take advantage of this opportunity to start a lifestyle change of your own along with the patient then:

If you have been sedentary for several years, or, if you are over 35 years of age, or, if you have any chronic illness for which you are being regularly followed by a medical advisor, talk it over with him or her. If you fall into any of the above categories or haven't had a complete physical examination in the past few years, you should get a thorough physical evaluation. Your medical advisor should be aware of this program and your participation in it. He or she should help you to set realistic and safe goals for yourself and help you to monitor your progress toward those goals. If there are circumstances regarding your personal health status that dictate abridgments and adjustments in this program, only your personal medical advisor is qualified to help you make those abridgments and adjustments.

Any exercise program you enter into should be started slowly, especially if you have been sedentary for a long period of time. This program is no exception, but if you follow it, you'll see results in a surprisingly short time. Though changing you nutritional habits and practices should help you to improve your health and fat to lean body mass ratio and help you to find and approach your ideal body weight, it won't do it alone. Exercise must be a part of your new lifestyle. Exercise is vital to your good health.

The human body is very adaptable, an important survival characteristic in most situations, but it works against you when it comes to trying to reduce your body fat by nutritional change only. This adaptability is why so many dieters fail when they try to lose weight by cutting caloric intake alone. We humans are a part of the animal kingdom and therefore we respond physiologically to starvation like most other animals. When other animals go into a starvation period, such as during famines or hibernation, their bodies go into conservation mode. Their metabolism is dramatically slowed to conserve fat stores. The same happens when the human animal starves itself during a diet. As soon as our bodies sense that they are being deprived of their usual quantity of food, the caloric intake we have become accustomed to, our systems slow down our metabolic rate—go into a very high efficiency mode—to preserve our storage fat. This adds to the dieter's frustration by slowing the rate of his or her weight loss and reduction of fat deposits.

> Othniel Seiden is an MD. His is a doctor,
> but he is not *your* doctor...
> You should ALWAYS consult
> with your physcian about
> lifestyle changes such as these.

Vigorous exercise helps to "override" our starvation defense system. Because exercise demands energy it forces our metabolic rate to remain high. Our bodies can't go into starvation or hibernation mode. Thus it is vitally important to exercise along with any nutritional changes we make in our eating habits to potentiate our burning off of body storage fat and toning and building of lean muscle mass—i.e., improving our fat to lean mass ratio and helping us approach our ideal body weight; and since muscle mass burns calories about thirty to forty times more than fat, even at rest, our metabolic rate is dramatically elevated so that we continue to burn more calories even after we are done exercising.

In addition to what exercise does to help us attain our ideal body weight, recent studies have shown that exercise is essential to prolonged life. Statistics now show conclusively that *even minimal exercise reduces premature death from all causes.* Let me repeat that statement. Even minimal exercise reduces premature death from all causes!

We have long advocated exercise to strengthen the cardiovascular system to reduce premature death from heart disease, but now strong evidence shows that exercise also reduces the rate of premature death from cancer, stroke, diabetes and apparently all other disease processes and normal causes of early death. And although the exact mechanism by which exercise will prolong life is not fully understood, it only makes sense that a physically fit body will resist illness, injury and heal faster and more completely when illness or injury does occur.

So what is moderate exercise? You will benefit by as little exercise as forty-five minutes of brisk walking three times a week. But for this program, I want you work yourself up to doing a very brisk walk an hour a day, five to seven days a week. That may sound rough to you right now, especially if you've been a sedentary person in the recent past, but it will pay off in more ways than you can imagine. Once you get into your workout program you won't think it tough at all. In the next chapter, we will work you into your exercise program and you'll be back into good physical condition amazingly soon.

If you've been a sedentary person, the idea of starting an exercise program may be intimidating to you. You see all those folks out there jogging, running marathons, biking, playing tennis, racquet ball and participating in triathlons—well you say you want no part of all that pain and effort. I've got good news for you. **The "no pain, no gain" bit is a myth.** The exercise program this book advocates is based strictly on walking. That's not to say you can't participate in other exercise activities. On the contrary, we advocate you participate in as many exercise or athletic activities as you desire, but, other activities do not replace your walking program. *Walking is an absolute must!* Regardless of whatever other activities you participate in, none can replace your walking program for its absolute perfect benefit to you physically, mentally and aerobically! This statement will be fully explained and defended in the next chapter. **The fact is**

that walking is humankind's most perfect aerobic exercise and by itself is all the exercise you need to become and stay physically fit for the rest of your life. Other exercise activities can benefit you in other ways but none can replace a good walking program for total conditioning; not biking, swimming, running, jogging, tennis, racquet ball, aerobic dance or calisthenics. Only cross country skiing is potentially better for you than a walking program, but only if you live where you can cross country ski daily the year around.

A walking program has the additional advantage of being accessible to everyone almost anywhere. It requires no special equipment, club membership, expensive investment, special clothing other than comfortable shoes. Special athletic skills are not a requirement.

If you are one of the rare individuals who has an illness that prevents brisk walking then we will suggest alternative aerobic activities for you in the next chapter.

For those of you who might be skeptical of the benefits of walking as your sole (no pun intended) exercise program, consider the following:

1. Walking is humankind's most natural exercise at any age. Of all exercises other than swimming or pool aerobics, it is the safest and least traumatic to body and joints. However, it is far more aerobic than both those low impact activities. We've been designed to walk great distances at remarkable speeds. Running was meant only for short spurts during the hunt or emergencies. We weren't designed or built to withstand the punishment of long continuous running or jogging which require lifting the body weight completely off the ground and landing on bent knees with each jarring stride.

2. Walking will exercise the entire body and mind. It utilizes the upper body more than running and the legs far more than swimming. In a vigorous, brisk walk there is virtually no muscle group in your body at rest. And as you will learn later on, walking stimulates mental and creative activity as well as reducing distress.

3. Walking will develop your endurance within safe boundaries faster than any other aerobic sport. No other sport can provide you with the benefits you will be getting from your walking program in as short a time as a week from now.

4. Your walking program will give you the best cardiovascular/cardiopulmonary (aerobic) workout you can get and with the greatest margin of safety.

5. Walking can be done by virtually anyone, anytime, anywhere. It is probably the most indulged in sport in the world. Over 40% of Americans will tell you that walking is their main source of exercise—and Americans are newcomers to the sport.

6. Walking is a family sport, one of the few that all ages can participate in equally, together.

7. We call walking a sport because it is a competitive event, even to the Olympic level, should you want to pursue it. Race walking is becoming popular throughout the United States as it has been in other parts of the world for decades. Competition is usually broken down into age groups so competition can be pursued at all ages into the eighties and older. Races are also divided into men's and women's divisions and are usually broken

down into 5, 10, 30 and 50 kilometer events. It is interesting to note that an Olympic or World Class race walker is among the best conditioned of all athletes.

8. If you're not interested in that kind of competition—and most of us aren't—the competition you'll have against yourself will be all you need to keep you going toward ever increasing goals.

9. You'll probably burn more calories, exercise your heart, lungs and circulation better, lose more weight and develop your body and mind further than you could in any other activity. In addition, walking will lower your blood pressure, reduce stress and cholesterol levels and take off up to one pound of fat a week even if you don't alter your eating habits.

Does that sound too good to be true? You've heard nothing yet! The book <u>HEALTHWALK</u>, by Bob Carlson and O.J. Seiden, MD (you already like **his** books); Fulcrum, Inc.; **ISBN # 1-55591-028-9**, lists the following as benefits of walking:

1. It reduces the likelihood of cardiovascular and cerebrovascular disease by increasing collateral circulation, the blood flow and size and tone of the vessels.

2. It strengthens the muscles of the body including the heart muscle and makes them work more efficiently.

3. It slows the heart rate by increasing the stroke volume, the volume of blood the heart is able to pump with one contraction.

4. It tends to reduce the height to which arterial pressure rises during exercise and stress.

5. It encourages the development of collateral circulation to the heart muscle. This can dramatically increase your chances of surviving a coronary occlusion were it to happen.

6. It reduces depositing of storage fat throughout the body.

7. It improves digestion and elimination of body wastes.

8. It increases the oxygen supply to the brain and increases mental sharpness. It potentiates creative thought processes and there is growing evidence that it prevents or slows development of Alzheimer's disease.

9. It tends to retard the aging process and gives a more youthful appearance.

10. It aids lymphatic circulation and blood circulation in general.

11. It stimulates the metabolism and the effect continues burning calories for hours after the cessation of exercise.

12. It increases respiratory capacity and aerobic power.

13. It benefits body growth and recovery from trauma.

14. It reduces blood fat or triglyceride levels.

15. It reduces insomnia and provides for better relaxation.

16. It reduces the incidence of minor illnesses, allergies, headaches and abdominal problems.

17. It improves coordination by activating neurotransmitter and training muscle fibers.

18. It increases flexibility of the joints and muscles and thus reduces aches and pains in the back, neck, and other body joints.

19. It circulates more oxygen to all body tissues.

20. It creates a better balance between oxygen required by the tissues and the oxygen made more readily available through exercise.

21. It tones up the glandular systems and increases thyroid gland output.

22. It increases the production of red blood cells by the bone marrow.

23. It increases the ability to store and utilize reserve nutrients which increases endurance.

24. It augments the alkaline reserve of the body which can be significant in an emergency requiring extended effort.

25. It gives a feeling of muscular strength by toning all the body muscles.

26. It counteracts feelings of fatigue.

27. It augments a chemical action which increases the potential of body cells.

28. It causes muscles to move vital fluids throughout the body which in turn lessens the work done by the heart.

29. It has a stabilizing effect on blood pressure and normalizes it.

30. It releases the flow of endorphin which is the body's own tranquilizer.

31. It has a hardening and strengthening effect on bones of the entire skeletal system.

32. It provides a reserve of body strength and physical efficiency.

33. It betters the ratio between high density and low density components of cholesterol which lessens the risk of artery disease and many cancers.

34. It greatly improves mental outlook, optimism, morale and self esteem.

35. It will even improve your sexual functioning and that's no small reward!

So there you are. With all that walking can do for you, you can't help but improve your physical and mental status and well being, The time to begin turning your life around is now. Step number one is to speak with your personal medical advisor and discuss your intentions with him or her. Take this book with you and get his or her input. Let him or her help you to set some realistic goals.

Now start walking!

CHAPTER 4

AEROBICS... YOUR CARDIOVASCULAR WORKOUT....

Let's start talking about "healthy!"

We've said already that walking is the best aerobic exercise you can participate in. You might at this point ask, "What is an *aerobic* exercise?" *Aerobic* means "with air" and refers to an activity that can be sustained without getting breathless—as opposed to *anaerobic*, which creates an oxygen debt and its resulting breathlessness. Aerobic exercise, as opposed to anaerobic exercise, utilizes maximum oxygen. It works the heart and lungs for longer periods at a time than anaerobic. Anaerobic tend to work muscles against resistance for short spurts of time and uses minimum amounts of oxygen.

Exercise physiologists have shown that to get maximum benefit from an aerobic exercise program you must maintain your ideal exercise pulse rate for 45 minutes and preferably for one hour. In addition to this you should do enough exercise to burn off at least 2,000 calories a week by exercising at least five and if possible seven days a week. Keeping these facts in mind, walking is the best, and in most cases, the only exercise to fill these requirements. There are very few, if any, other exercises most of us can keep up for 45 minutes, much less for a full hour, while maintaining our ideal exercise pulse rate. But by brisk walking most of us can accomplish just that. If you can't do it now, you will be able to in just a few weeks of conditioning.

When you walk a mile on level ground, regardless of the speed in which you do it, you will burn off about 100 Calories. Thus, if you walk four miles in one hour, you'll be burning off 400 Calories each day and in only five days will burn your 2,000 Calorie weekly quota. If you walk six or seven days, that's all the better. And if you walk a full hour you'll be maintaining your ideal exercise pulse rate for over 45 minutes, even allowing for a warm up and cool down period. I can think of no other exercise that so perfectly meets all these physiological criteria for a good aerobic workout.

Now let's determine YOUR IDEAL EXERCISE PULSE RATE. Your personal rate is determined by your age. The formula is as follows:

220 minus your age times .70

Thus, if your age is 65 years old, your ideal exercise pulse rate would be:

$$220 - 65 = 155$$
$$155 \times .70 = 108$$

Your ideal exercise pulse rate would be 108 beats per minute. In other words, you would want to walk at a speed that would maintain your pulse at 108 beats per minute for 45 minutes to one hour.

There are three other pulse rate figures you should know about; *your minimum exercise pulse rate—your maximum exercise pulse rate and your resting pulse rate.*

Your minimum exercise pulse rate =
220 - your age X .60
Your maximum exercise pulse rate =
220 - your age X .80

Thus, if you are 65 years of age your minimum exercise pulse rate would be 155 X .60 = 93 beats per minute and your maximum exercise pulse rate would be 155 X .80 = 124 beats per minute.

What these figures mean to you is that if you are walking so slow that your pulse rate is less than your minimum exercise pulse rate, it is doing you little aerobic good. If you are walking so fast that your pulse is beating faster than your maximum exercise pulse rate, you should slow your pace enough to drop below that number. So if you are indeed 65 years of age you should try to walk fast enough to keep your pulse between 100 and 120 beats per minute for 45 minutes to an hour, preferably at 108 to 115 beats per minute.

Before we talk about resting pulse rate, find your minimum, maximum and ideal exercise pulse rates on the line with your age in the table. Memorize them.

RESTING PULSE RATE.

The importance of your resting pulse rate is that it is one of the best measures of your cardiovascular improvement as you progress in your walking program. To determine your resting pulse rate, take it first thing upon waking in the morning before you get out of bed. If you can't take it then, count it after sitting or lying down completely relaxed for about ten minutes. Try to take it at the same time and under the same conditions each day. As you get into better condition, your resting pulse will become lower and lower. Other measures of your improvement are discussed in the chapter, **Weights and Measures**.

Now let's get back to your exercise goal—*to develop your cardiovascular/cardiopulmonary health so you can walk an hour at your own ideal exercise pulse rate*—thus achieving and maintaining your best fitness potential.

Decide *with your physician* what your beginning level of

AGE	MINIMAL E.P.R	IDEAL E.P.R.	MAXIMUM E.P.R.
20-30	114-120	133-140	152-160
30-40	108-114	125-133	144-152
40-50	102-108	119-125	136-144
50-55	99-102	115-119	132-136
55-60	96-99	112-115	128-132
60-65	93-96	108-112	124-128
65-70	90-93	105-108	120-124
70-75	87-90	101-105	116-120
75-80	84-87	98-101	112-116
80-85	81-84	94	108-112
85-90	78-81	91-94	104-108
90 PLUS	75	90	104

exercise should be. If in doubt, start out with a minimal walk. Do what you know you can do, even if it is only a few steps. If you do it with more ease than you expected, then add a few more steps with each walk you take. Even if you're just getting out of a sick bed and your walks are only a few feet, do them as often in the day as you can. Your walking program will progress at a much faster pace than you can imagine. Until you can walk for twenty minutes without a stop, don't feel you have to push yourself too far beyond comfort. The important thing is to make each walk a little further and/or a little faster than the last. And walk every day. Make it part of your daily routine, preferably at the same time each day. It has to be scheduled to give it its proper priority among all the other things you do each day, then schedule it. In fact, it has to be at the very top of your priorities. Realize, **any day you don't find time to exercise walk, you're saying everything you do that day is more important than your health!** Your health is your most important asset!

To help you measure your progress, record on paper how far you walk each day and how long it takes you. At the end of each week compare and chart your progress. You'll be amazed at the rapid improvement. There are tables to record your progress at the end of this book.

When you finally get to the point where you can walk a full hour non-stop—and it will happen sooner than you (or your doctor) think—you should start to increase your pace a little each day until you reach your ideal exercise pulse rate. Once you reach that level, it does not mean you won't improve any more. Your physical condition will still improve gradually and you'll notice it because you'll have to walk faster over time to get your heart rate up to your ideal exercise level. Thus you ideal exercise pulse rate will become another measure of your continuing cardiopulmonary health development along with your resting pulse rate.

Let's review the other measures of your gains in physical health:

1. You will feel better all over with fewer aches and pains. When something does bother you you'll bounce back quicker. You'll probably have fewer "down days."

2. You'll look far better, having more muscle tone throughout your entire body. You may not lose much weight, but you'll have less fat and look trimmer.

3. You'll be happier, more confident, have more

energy and interests. Your friends and family will notice.

4. You'll sleep better, deeper, more soundly.

5. You'll find your joints are more supple and limber and less subject to pain, injury and stiffness. Movement will be more fluid and easier.

6. You'll think better, clearer and more creatively because of the improved circulation to your brain. This will impact the efficiency with which you do your job.

7. You'll want to get out and do things you thought you'd never be interested in again. You'll want to get out and do things.

8. You'll enjoy friends and relatives a lot more and they'll enjoy you. All your relationships should improve.

9. You'll stop feeling sorry for yourself and may well want to help others achieve your state of health and happiness for themselves.

10. You'll start looking for and setting new goals for yourself.

11. You'll start thinking of your bright future instead of living in the past—realizing that your life is still very much in front of you.

So get up *right now* and take your first steps toward that new life in front of you!

A lot has been written about stretching and warming up before you exercise. **The best warm up for walking is walking.** Spend the first four or five minutes of your walk gradually working up to your best exercise pace. Start out at a comfortable walk and gradually increase your stride and speed until you fall into a brisk rhythm that is adequate to give you a good cardiovascular workout.

More important than the warm up to your walk is an adequate cool down period at the end of your walk. *Never, never* just stop after you've been walking at your ideal exercise pulse rate or faster without cooling down with a slower walk. Reduce you speed and continue to walk until your pulse is slowed to under your minimal exercise rate or less than 100, whichever is lower.

Then if you want, do some stretching exercises. Do them *after* your workout. It is amazing how often people injure themselves by overstretching while their muscles are cold and tight before their workout. If you start your walk slow and easy and build up your pace, the muscles will warm up and limber safely. Then do your stretching after the vigorous workout. You will get all the benefits of stretching without the danger of injury. Furthermore, the post exercise stretching will keep you from getting stiff and painful muscles and joints after too vigorous a workout.

What about other sports? And what if you can't walk?

As for those few of you who can't walk due to a real physical handicap, the same principles apply. You must find an activity that will keep your pulse rate at its ideal exercise level for 45 minutes to an hour. Consider swimming, rowing or bicycling on a stationary rowing machine or bike or other water exercises such as pool aerobics, or just walk back and forth in a pool, trying to increase your speed and distance. You may find that these exercises will improve your condition to where you will be able to work into a walking program after all.

For those of you confined to a wheel chair, 45 minutes to an hour of wheeling yourself around a park is an ideal workout. Begin the same as recommended for the walking program, an easy spin at first, gradually adding to your time and distance and then adding to your speed until your working at your ideal exercise pulse rate for 45 minutes to an hour. You may even work up to where you can compete in races or other wheel chair sports.

If you are bedridden or otherwise confined by your physical health, ask your physician about a physical therapy consultation to determine your true potential and how to reach it. There are very few who can do no exercise, but for those few, you can still maximize your fitness and life span by following the other lifestyle changes recommended in this book.

As for other exercises and sports activities, they are great if you enjoy them, but they do not replace your walking program. You should participate in as many exercise or athletic activities as you enjoy, over and above your walking program. On the other hand, you need no other exercise activities other than your walking program if you don't want to do any more. It is a good idea to have some other aerobic exercises available to you for those days when you can't walk because of inclement weather or some other preventing problem. Swimming, stationary biking or rowing are all ideal. All are good aerobic, low impact activities.

Such activities as tennis, racquet ball, baseball, weight lifting and training or body building, are anaerobic and wonderful activities, if you enjoy them, but remember they do not take the place of your walking program and must be done in addition to your walking. Golf and bowling are great social and stress reducing activities and help keep your joints limber, but are neither anaerobic nor aerobic. Again, if you enjoy them, participate in them in addition to your walking program.

A special note about weight lifting and body building; both of these activities put special stresses on the heart and vascular system which may have a detrimental effect on some cardiovascular conditions. Be sure to get a clearance and limitation of these activities from your cardiologist or cardiovascular surgeon!

And don't forget that daily chores are also calorie burners. Don't farm them out to others to benefit from the activities. Do your own gardening, yard work, minor repairing. Below is a list of calorie expenditures for various activities. Just sitting on the couch burns few calories.

Exercise Calorie Burners by Various Activities

This table will give you a rough idea of how many calories you may be burning at various activities when performed for 30 minutes. The caloric expenditure listed is for a person of 100, 150, 200 and 300 pounds. Your weight will probably fall between the columns, requiring you to guestimate your approximate caloric expenditure. Depending on how vigorous the exercise, you can add or subtract between 10 and 20 calories for every ten pounds you weigh over or under the columns surrounding your actual weight. This is one place us heavy weights get a break; we actually burn more Calories than skinny folks!

Exercise is extremely important to cardiac patients. When my father had his first heart attack or coronary occlusion over forty years ago, he was told to reduce his activity drastically. He had to move his bedroom from the second to the first floor to avoid steps. He was told to stay at bed rest for weeks, both in the hospital and after he got home a month and a half after his myocardial infarction. When he was allowed to resume activity he was warned not to exert himself—ever! That was how heart disease was treated in those days. When Othniel went to

ACTIVITY	100 LBS	150 LBS	200 LBS	300 LBS
Aerobic dancing (low impact)	115	172	230	345
Aerobics step training, 4" step (beginner)	145	218	290	435
Aerobics, slide training (basic)	150	225	300	435
Backpacking with 10 lb. load	180	270	360	540
Backpacking with 20 lb. load	200	300	400	600
Backpacking with 30 lb. load	235	352	470	705
Badminton	150	225	300	450
Basketball (game)	220	330	440	660
Basketball (leisurely, nongame)	130	195	260	390
Bicycling, 10 mph (6 minutes/mile)	125	188	250	375
Bicycling, 13 mph (4.6 minutes/mile)	200	300	400	600
Billiards	45	68	90	135
Bowling	55	82	110	165
Canoeing, 2.5 mph	70	105	140	210
Canoeing, 4.0 mph	135	202	270	405
Croquet	60	90	120	180
Cross country snow skiing, intense	330	495	660	990
Cross country snow skiing, leisurely	155	232	310	465
Cross country snow skiing, moderate	220	330	440	660
Dancing (noncontact)	100	150	200	300
Dancing (slow)	55	82	110	165
Gardening, moderate	90	135	180	270
Golfing (walking, w/o cart)	100	150	200	300
Golfing (with a cart)	70	105	140	210

Handball	230	345	460	690
Hiking with a 10 lb. load	180	270	360	540
Hiking with a 20 lb. load	200	300	400	600
Hiking with a 30 lb. load	235	352	470	705
Hiking, no load	155	232	310	465
Housework	90	135	180	270
Ironing	50	75	100	150
Jogging, 5 mph (12 minutes/mile)	185	278	370	555
Jogging, 6 mph (10 minutes/mile)	230	345	460	690
Mopping	85	128	170	255
Mowing	135	202	270	405
Ping Pong	90	135	180	270
Raking	75	112	150	225
Raquetball	205	308	410	615
Rowing (leisurely)	75	112	150	225
Rowing machine	180	270	360	540
Running, 08 mph (7.5 minutes/mile)	305	458	610	915
Running, 09 mph (6.7 minutes/mile)	330	495	660	990
Running, 10 mph (6 minutes/mile)	350	525	700	1050
Scrubbing the floor	140	210	280	420
Scuba diving	190	285	380	570
Shopping for groceries	60	90	120	180
Skipping rope	285	428	570	855
Snow shoveling	195	292	390	585
Snow skiing, downhill	130	195	260	390

Soccer	195	292	390	585
Squash	205	308	410	615
Stair climber machine	160	240	320	480
Stair climbing	140	210	280	420
Swimming (25 yards/minute)	120	180	240	360
Swimming (50 yards/minute)	225	338	450	675
Table Tennis	90	135	180	270
Tennis	160	240	320	480
Tennis (doubles)	110	165	220	330
Trimming hedges	105	158	210	315
Vacuuming	75	112	150	225
Volleyball (game)	120	180	240	360
Volleyball (leisurely)	70	105	140	210
Walking, 2 mph (30 minutes/mile)	60	90	120	180
Walking, 3 mph (20 minutes/mile)	80	120	160	240
Walking, 4 mph (15 minutes/mile)	100	150	200	300
Washing the car	75	112	150	225
Waterskiing	160	240	320	480
Waxing the car	100	150	200	300
Weeding	100	150	200	300
Weight training (40 sec. between sets)	255	382	510	765
Weight training (60 sec. between sets)	190	285	380	570
Weight training (90 sec. between sets)	125	188	250	375
Window cleaning	75	112	150	225

medical school a decade later, they still advocated inactivity for heart patients. Sad to say, we were not curing heart disease, we were creating **cardiac cripples.**

Today we know better. The heart is a muscle. And like any muscle of the body it improves and strengthens with *prudent exercise.* Most importantly, the increased circulation of blood provides increased oxygen to nourish its hungering muscle cells. Think about this; in most cases, it is a sedentary lifestyle that causes heart disease. It is thus unlikely that a sedentary lifestyle will improve your cardiac status.

Prudent exercise, on the other hand, can prevent heart disease—and it will in most cases improve dramatically an already diseased or damaged heart. So what do we mean by, *"Prudent exercise?"* First of all, it must be designed for you specifically! This means supervision and approval of your physician; careful adherence to the prescribed program by you, and consideration of all points covered in the following pages. It is strongly recommended that you take this book with you when you discuss your mending heart fitness program with your medical advisor, so there will be no misunderstanding of what is intended by either of you. Talk to your physician about working out in a cardiac rehab program to get you started in the right direction and to create a program fir you.

The exercise you need to improve your heart is an aerobic program. An aerobic exercise is one which causes you to breathe deeply and increase your pulse rate to *your ideal exercise pulse rate for a prolonged time*—eventually 45 minutes to one hour per day. The purpose of an aerobic exercise program is to build cardiovascular and cardiopulmonary strength and endurance; in other words, to strengthen your heart, lungs and circulatory system so they will function most efficiently and have adequate reserve in distressful and emergency situations.

Most heart disease patients should be able to adopt and adapt to this program with minimal difficulty and in a short time resume the most active, productive, confident, healthy, happy life he or she has ever known.

And the goal of this book is to help you become the most fit that you can possibly be, to become the most active, productive, confident, healthy, happy, you that you can be—perhaps have ever been!

You needn't walk more than four miles a day, and in some cases, not even that far. The time you spend walking is far more important than the actual distance. We're going to set your sights on eventually walking one hour a day. Think you can't do an hour a day? Well, if you don't have a physically crippling defect that keeps you from walking, you can probably very easily walk an hour a day. It is probably not a matter of physical inability but a matter of priority. Believe it, your health is well worth an hour a day. Busier people than you have found the time—so can you. You must if you want to reach your life potential.

MORE ABOUT AEROBICS FOR PEOPLE WITH LIMITED MOBILITY

Fortunately, there are numerous practical options some of which we've mentioned; let's look in some more detail.

Swimming and pool exercise...

For a person with limited mobility, water exercises may prove ideal for several reasons, because it presents a range of resistance to the muscles with markedly reduced weight bearing. In some cases, you can even use a walker or special wheelchair in the exercise pool. There are counter current pools available for installation in private residences or apartment and condominium facilities where you adjust the water current flow so you can swim in place or walk with a specific measured challenge.

Water walking can be an excellent option for people with weight bearing problems or arthritic hip, knee or ankle joints. By using a pool noodle, a buoyant foam tube, under your arms or buttock while in the water, you can actually float in one place while moving your legs as though walking, thus getting considerable aerobic benefits. A person who can't swim or has mobility handicaps must exercise in water with caution and never go in a pool unsupervised. You might also consider wearing a life jacket or an AquaJogger, a buoyant strap on belt to make you safer in the water. In most areas, water aerobic classes are readily available.

If you can swim at all, try working up to swimming 30 minutes to an hour a day or at least three times a week. Think you can't do that? Most people are limited to short distances swimming by their ability to coordinate their breathing. If that's your problem, try swimming with a snorkel. That will let you breath without having to bring your head out of the water and you will find you can swim what seems almost indefinitely, but for sure 30 to 60 minutes. Swimming is an excellent upper body and endurance builder. Combining swimming with other water exercises burns calories at a high rate and is very aerobic.

Bicycles stationary or mobile...

Stationary bicycles are readily available to the mobility-challenged person who retains the ability to move his or her legs. They come in two main styles, the most common configured like a normal bike or a recumbent style which is more comfortable for someone who as difficulty sitting in a saddle type seat. If one is able to ride a regular bike but has difficulty bearing weight for prolonged periods, a standard bike may work quite well.

Arm only aerobics for those with upper body ability only...

Even if you have absolutely no use of your legs, aerobic exercise is still within your reach. An arm ergometer, a device which looks almost like an inverted stationary bicycle, is available in clubs or for home use. The user sits facing peddles, but grasps them with his or her hands rather than peddling with the feet. They rotate exactly like a bicycle but are powered by your arms providing excellent aerobic exercise.

In addition, there are numerous seated circulation workouts, seated weight workouts and some leg strengthening exercises that might require standing but not walking. Exercise leaders are available on DVD or easily followed programs on TV. Of course, for people still able to walk even just a few steps, it's possible to get a significant workout using walkers or wheelchairs as mentioned before. If you are easily tired out, concentrate on short exercise intervals and repeat several times a day building up your endurance.

In all cases, it is important that if you're of limited mobility always discuss your exercise plans with your health-care professional.

If you think you're unable to exercise, consider my mother in law who had open heart surgery to replace a defective heart valve when she was 83 years old. In addition, she had a cardiac pacemaker installed. For at least two decades before her surgery, she hadn't walked more than 100 feet at a time without sitting down for a prolonged rest. Within two days of her surgery, we started her on her walking program. It started with a walk from her bed to the bathroom less than ten feet away. The next day, we walked her out into the hall a few feet, to a chair, and then back to her bed. She did that four times that day and it exhausted her. The next day, we walked her in the hospital hall for about 50 feet and back to the chair, and after a brief rest another 50 foot walk and back to bed. We did that routine about six times that day. The next day she did about 100 feet of hallway about ten different times. She was surprised to discover that was about a fifth of a mile.

Her walks increased daily and by the time she left the hospital ten days post surgery, she was doing about a mile a day in the halls of the hospital in divided doses. She left the hospital about five days earlier than her surgeon expected her to and he credited her rapid recovery on her daily forced walks.

When we got her home she started walking outside or in shopping centers when the weather was too inclement. Within four weeks of her hospital discharge, she was walking an hour non-stop and clipping off three miles, or a mile every twenty minutes. That's a very comfortable and easy pace for most people. Today she walks a mile in 16 to 17 minutes with surprising ease for a 90 year old. She walks four miles a day six or seven days a week with a proud bounce to her stride and is healthier and more active than she's been in the past thirty years. **And when the weather is good—she plays 9 holes of golf a week "with the girls!"**

Set your goals in her footsteps!

Discuss your walking plans with your personal medical advisor. Show him or her this book and decide at what level you should begin—and then begin—today! If it's from your bed to the toilet and back, so be it. If you can walk a few hundred feet in the hall, so be it. If you can walk a mile, however slow, great! So be it! Wherever you can start—start—but start today! And if it goes well today, then go a bit further tomorrow, and a bit further each succeeding day until you can walk an hour. And when you can walk an hour a day, pick up the speed a little each day, which will lengthen the distance of your one hour walk each day. And continue picking up the speed of your walk until you reach *your ideal exercise pulse rate.* Then as your general health and cardiac and pulmonary fitness improve, you will be able to walk faster and further in that hour while maintaining your ideal exercise pulse rate; *for now do what you can do comfortably!*

Chapter 5

You Really "Are What You Eat!"

It is amazing that the tremendous increase in nutritional knowledge our scientists have accumulated in the past decade has just supported the correctness of the diet our long lived primitive counterparts have been eating for centuries.

These simple diets have not come about by insight or wisdom, but because of what has been provided for them by nature and tradition. The similarity in their foods is remarkable even though they live worlds apart. Interesting is the fact that until the Japanese had their diet westernized by our influence since World War II, they also didn't have the heart problems, cancers, strokes, diabetes and terminal diseases we have. Since their diet changed to emulate ours and we began exporting our smoking habits to them, their death rates from these illnesses have rocketed to our levels; proof that our eating and smoking habits are killers.

Now that we've started on an exercise program to put our cardiovascular systems into better aerobic fitness, let's bring our nutrition into a life preserving mode. Not only will the foods you eat from now on lengthen your life, but they will keep you as physically fit as possible to promote energy for activity and reduce many of the joint and muscle problems that put too many of our elderly into rocking chairs and wheel chairs.

Now let's get one other thing straight; this book isn't telling fat Greyhounds not to become thin Greyhounds. If you happen to be one of those five percent who can take it off and keep it off, go for it. But if you've been yo-yoing your weight up and down for the past decade or two, it's time to try a new approach. **Folks who are destined to be heavy can indeed be healthy.*** Weight is only one factor in our total health profile, and if you can get the other factors in line, *your weight makes little difference.*

* Heavy and Healthy - ISBN: 0-9779960-5-0

Let me also underline that **diets rarely work**. Oh, you may knock off 20, 25, 30 or even much more weight on one diet or another, but as soon as you go off of it, you'll gain back 25, 35, 45 or much more weight than you originally lost. Sound familiar? It should. Remember, national averages show that less than ten percent of all of us ever keep off the weight we took off on all the various diets we tried from time to time. The yo-yoing of our weight during and between diets is far unhealthier than the weight we originally wanted to take off. Almost all diets are fads. They are at best temporary. Most are dangerous to your health.

This book does not put you on a diet!

In fact, if you follow this *program* you'll never diet again! And, if you follow this program, *a year from today you'll be the best you can be—possibly the best you have ever been!* That's the goal of this book and program, to put you into the best condition you can be in, to catapult you into the second half of your life— to guarantee the maximum healthy, productive and pleasurable years of your 120 potential.

There are some of us, perhaps most of us, who are just not destined to be Madison Avenue gods and goddesses or match a predetermined spot on a weight chart. Neither the weight charts nor Madison Avenue are necessarily the best health standards for us to set our goals toward. And just because we don't match up—or rather down, to those arbitrary standards, does not mean we are any less valuable a person or are less healthy than the *skinny folks*. In fact, there is a real rebellion in the modeling industry now because there have been some unfortunate deaths among models because of their unhealthy efforts to maintain such unrealistic low weights.

In this book and program, we set more realistic weight and health standards for you. We'll forget weight charts, which were invented by an insurance company and not public health authorities or physicians—rather we will help you determine your own *Ideal Body Weight*. Ideal Body Weight is a concept that makes a lot more sense, is far more realistic and does not threaten your health in trying to attain it through every insane fad diet that comes along.

Over the past decade alone there have been hundreds, perhaps thousands of diet books published—and yet our population is probably more out of shape, obese and unhealthy than ever before. In this program, we only discuss only good nutrition. **You'll probably be surprised to discover that most overweight people are also malnourished.** If we can correct this malnourishment we've gone a long way to improving health and we begin to approach our own *personal Ideal Body Weight*.

No chart or beauty standard set by the marketing moguls of Madison Avenue can determine what *you as an individual should weigh*. That would be as ridiculous as Madison Avenue or some insurance company telling you what your personality, attitudes, life goals, likes and dislikes and all other traits that make us individuals, should be.

If after all those diets you've been on and off of, you finally realized that you're just destined to spend the rest of your life "portly" and weighing well over what those charts say you should weigh, then this program is still—perhaps especially—for you! This program will help you find that Ideal Body Weight which is yours and yours alone—and will help you to attain and maintain that weight and the best health you can possibly have. You can be both "HEAVY AND HEALTHY!" You'll be far healthier than if you continue to try to reach and maintain a weight that is plainly unrealistic for you with every insane, faddish, yo-yo diet that comes along.

And so, let's get on with it!

NEVER DIET AGAIN...

Let me reiterate, "The word diet is not part of this program or book!" In fact, **YOU SHOULD NEVER DIET AGAIN!** Dieting is usually unhealthy, unnatural and almost always a frustrating failure. Dieting usually is a precursor to further weight gain to an even higher level—and another unhealthy fad diet. Simply stated, **dieting is usually futile! THIS IS AN ANTI-DIET PROGRAM AND BOOK!**

The gist of this program is "Weight Control." You may not even need to lose weight to be the best that you can be and if your weight is too high, it may not need to come down nearly as much as you might suspect. Does that sound too good to be true? Well it's not! The problem that too many of us face is the weight standard is not established by health authorities, but rather by the Madison Avenue agencies, the fashion industry or a **self-serving** and **uninformed** insurance industry.

This program will help you to set new, proper, healthy, realistic and above all safe weight standards for yourself. And once set, it will show you how to achieve and maintain *your own ideal body weight.*

Let's summarize:

1. You are never going to diet again. For us the word "diet" no longer exists!

2. We are going to get as near our *individual Ideal Body Weight* and maintain it for life, be that Ideal Body Weight higher or lower than our present weight.

3. In addition to being *in control of our Ideal Body Weights*, a year from now, we will be in the best health and shape we can possibly attain.

Since we no longer recognize the word "d--t" we need a new concept—not a synonym for the word d--t—a concept with truly a different meaning. It's not a coined concept or new idea. It's a concept you've known since at least grade school, but we'll personalize it for you, make it palatable to you, make it work for you, make it easily understood by you. You, you, you.... You are the person who is the subject of this program. For it to succeed, it has to succeed for you. The concept that will make it work for you for the rest of your life to achieve and maintain *your* ideal body weight is—*simple good nutrition!*

Here the key word is simple. You needn't become a nutritionist. A few simple insights will let you select the best foods to satisfy your personal weight, nutritional and appetite needs.

Before we go any further let's set some realistic goals.

LONGEVITY...

The ultimate goal should be for a long and healthy life; an active life and a productive life. It is pointless to add years onto your life unless you can put happy life into those years. So let's set our first goal at living as many of our potential 120 years as humanly possible and enjoying them all to their fullest. Following are a few sub-goals that will make our main goal possible and worthwhile.

1. A year from today, you are to be the best that we can be physically and mentally—possibly the best we've ever been!

2. Once achieved, to maintain this excellent condition to your dying day—may you live to 120!

3. To enjoy every minute of those long and happy, healthy years.

Well, let's take on the nutritional challenge! We'll do it in stages, gradually, so as not to be overwhelmed. To start we'll make a few minor, painless changes in our nutrition...

DEFENSIVE SHOPPING....

Let's attack this problem a little differently. Our Third World friends don't eat better than we do because they're smarter than we are. They eat the way they do because nature has dealt them a kind hand. She's made the bad nutrition unavailable to them—put only the healthy things in their food sources. So let's take a lesson from nature. Instead of listing all the things we should and shouldn't eat, let's make the bad stuff unavailable. If it's not there we can't eat it. Thus, we should concentrate on defensive shopping. If you don't buy it, it won't be in your cupboard—and if it's not in the cupboard, you're not likely to eat it too often. Notice I said, "Too often," not, "Never!" Once in a while you're bound to bite into the wrong things—just don't let it be "too often!"

There are many things that influence our food selection when we shop. Recognizing them will help us to avoid stocking up on the wrong foods.

TRADITION...

Among the strongest selection forces as we shop are our ethnic background and family or cultural traditions. Nostalgia is a big factor in our shopping and eating habits. Just remembering how my grandmother made her apple strudel makes it difficult to pass up the pastry department without thinking about buying a desert that isn't going to help my weight problem one little bit. And even though there aren't too many bakeries that make a thin crust strudel like grandma did, the memory translates into apple turnovers, apple pie, apple tarts, apple Danish or anything else that smells and tastes of apples, cinnamon, nuts, raisins, butter, etc., etc., etc. And if there isn't that to get nostalgic about, there's always the great cheesecake my mom used to make!

Being of European and Jewish extraction, there are plenty of other things to wet my already too easily influenced appetite. Matzo ball soup, chopped liver, Polish sausage, corned beef, hot pastrami, Vienna pastries, Kaiser rolls, Hungarian pastries, herring in sour cream, cheeses, salami, sausages of all kinds, dumplings, goose—the list goes on and on and on and on. It's hard to walk through a modern day market without remembering those delicacies and not buy and buy and buy. That later translates into eat and eat and eat.

But there are also other fond memories; beet borscht, gefilte fish, roast chicken and turkey, good rye bread, lean boiled chicken or beef, baked fish, poached fish, smoked fish, all kinds of stews, hot vegetable soup—and that list goes on and on and on also.

The second list is a bit healthier than the first. And the point is not that I'll never eat from the first list again. But I'll fill my shopping cart from list two and save the occasional item from list one for special occasions. They become that much more pleasant if they aren't an everyday event. A once-in-a-while delicatessen lunch out becomes a heavenly experience.

I've listed the items that turn my appetite on and you'll have your own lists. The idea is for you to divide up between what's alright to have in your home and what to keep out—except for not-too-frequent special occasions. After you learn how to select healthy foods to keep in your home you'll find there will still be plenty of items to let you keep up the family, cultural and ethnic traditions your stomach has become fond of.

MARKETING...

Next to what you like, the succeeding strongest motivator of your buying habits is what your food market wants you to buy. Have you ever noticed that all those coupons and specials are rarely if ever for foods that are really good for you? There is a science and art to the way foods are displayed and marketed in the super markets. That arts and science of food marketing is aimed at only one thing, that's to get you to buy, buy and buy some more. It has no intention on making you buy what's good for you; it is aimed wholly on making you buy what is good for the super market's profit column. That's why when we go shopping, we invariably buy much more than we intended of items we had no notion of getting. How often have you gone into a store to pick up one ingredient you needed—say a dozen eggs—and came home with over $20.00 in food you really didn't need? The arts and science of "good" marketing did it to you. That's "good" marketing for the store!

> The most significant fact in all this is
> that as economic status increases,
> the food we eat
> tends to become less healthy.

ECONOMIC STATUS...

Think back to how you ate before you made it big. Our economic status has a lot to do with how we buy food. If you don't think so, go into a supermarket in a part of town that is a lower or higher economic status than where you live or usually shop. You'll be amazed at how differently even the same food chains will stock their stores in different areas of town. And as you might expect the prices on the same items will vary from area to area.

You won't easily find prime beef in poorer neighborhoods—and prime beef is much higher in fat and cholesterol than U.S. Good or Choice meats. Poorer areas will sell more chicken, beans, inexpensive fish, while the fancier neighborhood stores will sell more expensive sea foods, i.e.; lobster, shrimp, crab, shellfish, all of which are unhealthier than the cheaper fish. Part of the reason why many people in the Third World eat healthier than we do is that they can't afford many of the exotic foods that are less healthy. Again, I'm not suggesting you never eat a lobster or crab or shrimp or oyster again, but I am suggesting you keep those foods for those special occasions and eat the healthier foods on the more regular basis. And we'll show you there are plenty of healthy exotic foods you'll love.

Convenience is another unhealthy trend that the rich can better afford. Today the markets are full of pre-

prepared dinners and dishes. Read the labels on those foods and you'll see they are usually high in fats, salt, preservatives and other chemicals that are not that good for us. Nothing beats fresh foods prepared in your own kitchen where you can control all that goes into it—and you.

HABITS...

Our eating pattern and thus our buying pattern is dictated heavily by habit. Some of our eating habits are good. Some are bad. What I'm asking you to do is learn which habits are good and emphasize them and then add a few more good habits you can learn to love—and de-emphasize the bad ones, completely eliminating those you can learn to live without. The way we eat, our eating habits, determine how we buy, our buying habits. But the easiest way to change our eating habits is to change our buying habits. As I said before, "If it's not in the cupboard it will be tough for you to eat it!"

What we are going to do from now on is stock up our cupboards with good, tasty, fun and enjoyable food that also happens to be nutritiously healthy. That's what we mean by defensive shopping.

Just what do our Third World cousins who live so long eat?

Actually it's only partly what they eat. Just as important is what they don't eat. Let's take a look.

Because of their environment and economic circumstances they eat very little red meat—and what little red meat they do eat is usually very lean. Third World cattle just don't fatten up too well. Either they live on islands, in jungle, high in mountains where grazing is impractical or red meat is just too costly for their meager incomes. Whatever the reason, they get most of their meat protein from chicken and fish. Their red meat consumption is from the rare lamb, goat or pig slaughtered for very special celebrations. This translates into very low animal fat consumption and low saturated fat and cholesterol in their food chain.

In addition to low animal fat consumption, these people from primitive areas of the world tend toward relatively high fiber nutrition. Fruits and vegetables are a major part of their readily available provisions. They can often be home grown on small plots and require no refrigeration—can be stored without high technology methods. Many fruits grow wild and are available for the picking. These people do not have the equipment or the economy to afford the refining of grains. Thus they use whole grain wheat, rice, oats, maize and whatever other grains are available. They eat their fruits and vegetables raw or only slightly cooked so the fiber is not broken down in preparation. All these factors increase the roughage or fiber in their daily food consumption. Food additives are seldom in what they ingest.

Dairy product consumption is also minimized, not because they are so wise, but because economics dictate. These people eat relatively few eggs because it is more prudent to sell eggs or let them hatch into edible poultry. The goat milk that they get from their herds is better used in the production of cheeses which they can sell to those who are wealthier. Again, these factors tend to reduce the animal fat and cholesterol consumption of these peoples.

What is the overall effect of these factors?

Reduction of dietary animal fat translates into reduction of heart disease, hypertension and stroke. Increase of fiber consumption translates into reduction of cancer, blood sugar levels, atherosclerosis and arteriosclerosis and many other chronic health problems which plague our society. In fact, the diseases which are responsible for most of the deaths in the United States—heart disease, cancer, stroke, hypertension, diabetes, renal failure—are not frequently found in primitive areas of the world. Their nutrition is probably the major factor in this difference. Relatively simple changes in our nutrition could reduce and perhaps help us to eliminate these diseases from our society. Certainly if you and I make these changes in our own nutrition, we'll be reducing our chances of developing these dread diseases. Reduce the chances of developing the diseases that kill most Americans and we'll be taking a long step towards increasing our longevity to that 120 year potential of active, quality life.

So what should we avoid in the market to make our successful lifestyle change come about more easily?

Ways to Replace Healthy Foods for Bad.

The fresher a food is and the nearer it is to its natural state, the healthier it is for eating. Fresh berries, fruits, raw veggies, and nuts and are great replacements for most snack foods which are a major fat and calorie sources for most Americans. These above mentioned snack food substitutes will satisfy our cravings for the sweets and high fat and calorie crunchy snacks we too often crave. Whole raw vegetables have lots of vitamins and minerals and are high in good fiber, so choose green, red, orange and yellow vegetables and fruits for snacking. Keep them easily available to be convenient to your impulse snacking. When cooking them, it is best to steam thus retaining the most nutritional value. Be careful with sauces, which may be high in calories, fats and excess salts which can reduce their natural good qualities.

When indulging in pasta or baked good you should seek those made of whole grains or 100% whole wheat. Don't be fooled by labels saying, "Whole Wheat," instead of "100% Whole Wheat" or "100% Whole Grain." Avoid white breads and noodles made from white refined flour with much of the nutritional content removed. The high starch content in white bread will affect your blood sugar as quickly as raw sugar. Avoid all sugary snacks and pastries and exchange them for fresh fruits. Dried fruits have had much of their water removed and because of their shrinkage they are very high in sugars and calories. A handful of dried fruits will contain far more calories and sugar than a whole fresh fruit which will be far more filling.

When it comes to meats, shop for lean meats and think of menus that emphasize fish. The omega-3 essential fatty acids in deep cold water ocean fish are often deficient in our diets, so try to serve seafood two or three times per week. Baked fish and chicken are healthier than fried and lean meats like bison, venison or turkey are healthier than higher fat beef or pork. Processed lunch meats, hot dogs, bacon, and sausages have a lot of junk and fat that you don't really want to put into in your body. If really you love these meats as I do, look for healthier low fat and additive versions and those labeled **"Kosher."**

Drink lots of water as your main beverage. If you get tired of plain water, add a slice of lemon or lime to add a touch of flavor. Don't be fooled into buying expensive bottled water. There are few places in the United States where bottled water is safer or better than inexpensive tap water. Bottled water can cost you over $6.00 a gallon as compared to tap water which costs less than 0.01 penny a gallon, or $3.00 a gallon of gasoline.

Some of the bad eating habits we have to try to change can be more difficult than altering our menus. If you tend to eat because you are bored, sad, unhappy or even when you're happy, get a hobby, or better yet, go out and take a walk or exercise. Exercise will help you solve problems far better than snacking. If you snack in front of the TV stick to fruits and veggies, or better yet, watch less TV and exercise, read a book or get out and enjoy friends. If many or most of your meals are eaten in restaurants, you can save a fortune and eat at home more often where you control what goes into your meals. By all means, **avoid fast food**; think of fast food as "fast gain food!" Most important, pay attention to how big the portions you consume are. In general, Americans eat gigantic portions compared to the rest of the world. Keep the junk food like potato chips, tortilla chips, ice cream, and candy out of the house. Keep healthy snacks like fruits, crunchy vegetables with dips, or nuts handy.

In summary, eat lots of vegetables and fruits picking a rainbow of colors available maximizing healthy vitamins and variety. Utilize non-starchy vegetables such as spinach, carrots, broccoli, tomatoes, cabbage or green beans with meals, avoiding excessive potatoes, white rice or packaged processed vegetable side dishes. Choose whole grain foods. Avoid over processed grain products. Use brown rice or whole wheat spaghetti when serving pastas. Consider using dried beans and legumes such as kidney or pinto beans, peas and lentils into your meals. Turn to fish in your meals 2-3 times a week. If not fish, select lean meats, not prime. Use more chicken and turkey. Turn to non-fat dairy such as skim milk, non-fat yogurt and non-fat cheese. Drink more water and avoid soda, fruit punch, sweetened teas and other sugar-sweetened drinks. Cook with liquid oils in place of solid fats that are high in saturated and worse, transfats. Remember that fats are twice as high in calories as proteins or carbohydrates. Avoid high calorie snack foods and desserts like chips, cookies, cakes, and ice cream. Watch your portion sizes!

This is a brief listing of the things you should avoid and a few of their substitutes. It does not mean you can never eat the avoidable. But the less you stock the unhealthy items, the easier and sooner you'll get them out of your eating habit system. Eliminating these *most-common-less healthy* foods is a good start on your way to good nutrition. You'll learn how to select the best foods for you and your family and you'll begin to really rid yourself of harmful foods.

WHAT ABOUT VITAMINS AND MINERALS?

What exactly are vitamins and minerals and why are they so important? Vitamins and minerals are substances found in the foods we eat. Both are needed for our bodies to work properly, to grow and develop properly and to repair normally when things go wrong. The vitamins essential to our health have special roles to play. Vitamins are either fat soluble or water soluble. Fat-soluble vitamins can be stored in the fatty tissues in our body as-well-as in our liver until our body requires them, then they are called into action, taken to where they're needed. The fat-soluble vitamins are A, D, E, and K.

The water-soluble vitamins are different in that they can't be stored in our body and if they aren't used within a short time of ingestion they are excreted from the body usually by the kidneys in the urine. Thus, the water-soluble vitamins must be continually replaced. The water-soluble vitamins C, all of the B vitamins which are B1 or thiamin, B2 or riboflavin, , B6 or pyridoxine, , B12 or cobalamine, biotin, pantothenic acid, niacin and folic acid. Our body is unable to make vitamins. We are able to get the vitamins we need for good health from the foods available to us. But since we don't all always eat all the foods that contain these vitamins some of us need supplemental vitamins.

Let's take a closer look at the vitamins, what they do and where they are found in our food chain.

Vitamin A

This vitamin is essential for good eyesight, especially night vision and also color vision. This vitamin also helps proper growth and maintains healthy skin. Foods that are rich in vitamin A include, eggs, milk, cheeses, apricots, nectarines, cantaloupe, carrots, sweet potatoes, spinach among others. Vitamin A is one vitamin which can be overdosed so too much supplementation can be dangerous. It is unlikely to be overdosed from foods containing it.

The B Vitamins

As mentioned above, there is more than one B vitamin. To review the list, there are the vitamins B1, B2, B6, B12, niacin, folic acid, biotin, and pantothenic acid. The B vitamins are important for proper metabolism making energy available when and where the body needs it. This group of vitamins is essential in making red blood cells, which carry oxygen throughout the body. Foods rich in the B vitamins include, whole grains, such as wheat and oats, nuts, fish, seafood, poultry and meats, eggs, dairy products, milk, cheeses and yogurt, leafy green vegetables, beans and peas, citrus fruits, such as oranges, lemons, limes and grape fruit. Many cereals and breads are now enriched with B vitamins.

Vitamin C

This vitamin is important for keeping body tissues, such as gums, mucous membranes, skin and muscles in good health and promotes healing. Vitamin C also helps resist infection and illness. Some of the foods rich in vitamin C include citrus fruits, cantaloupe, strawberries, tomatoes, broccoli and cabbage.

Vitamin D

Vitamin D is needed for strong bones, necessary for the body to properly absorb and utilize calcium. It's also needed for formation and maintenance of strong teeth. There is some evidence that high doses of vitamin D may reduce allergies like hay fever. Foods rich in vitamin D include milk and other dairy products fortified with vitamin D, fish, egg yolks and though it isn't a food, about fifteen minutes of sunshine a day will satisfy most of our needs for Vitamin D. You'll get that on your walk...

Vitamin E

Vitamin E maintains your body's tissues, in your eyes, skin, and liver. **It protects your lungs from polluted air.** And it is important for the formation of red blood cells. Vitamin E is found prevalent in whole grains, wheat germ, leafy green vegetables, sardines, egg yolks and nuts.

Vitamin K

Vitamin K is essential for blood clotting. Foods are rich in vitamin K are leafy green vegetables, liver, pork and dairy products, like milk and yogurt

Minerals

Minerals are essential for life enabling normal cellular functions and metabolic reactions to occur. They maintain the structural integrity of the bones and facilitate the absorption of vitamins. The minerals, unlike vitamins, are not destroyed during food storage, cooking or processing. There are 16 minerals required for human life and they are divided into trace minerals, required in smaller quantity and macronutrients required in relatively larger quantities. The trace minerals include Chromium, Copper, Fluorine, Iodine, Iron, Manganese, Molybdenum, Selenium and Zinc. The major or macronutrient minerals are Calcium, Chloride, Magnesium, Phosphorus, Potassium, Sodium and Sulfur.

The American Dietetic Association provides the following information on minerals.

Calcium builds bones, both in length and strength, and prevents rapid bone loss as you age. It helps muscles contract, plays a role in normal nerve function, and helps blood coagulate when bleeding. **Deficiency** problems will affects bone density and increases the risk of osteoporosis and increases fragility leading to fractures. Foods rich in calcium include milk and milk products, some dark green leafy vegetables, fish with edible bones and tofu made with calcium. Many foods are fortified with calcium, such as some brands of orange juice, bread and soy milk. Excess calcium, over a prolonged period, can cause constipation, kidney stones and poor kidney function. It may also interfere with the absorption of other minerals, such as iron and zinc. Excess amounts are usually consumed through too much supplementation.

Phosphorus helps our body cells produce energy and is a major regulator of energy metabolism in our bodily organs. It is a major component of bones and teeth, and makes up part of our DNA and RNA. **Deficiency** is extremely rare, except in some premature babies who consume only breast milk, or for people taking aluminum hydroxide containing antacid over long periods of time. Symptoms include bone loss, weakness, loss of appetite and pain. **Food sources** include protein-rich food, legumes, nuts, bread and baked goods. Too much phosphorus may lower calcium levels in the blood and increase bone loss if calcium intake is insufficient.

Magnesium is an important part of more than 300 enzymes which regulate body functions, energy production and muscle contractions, along with maintaining nerve and muscle cells. It is also an important component of bones. **Deficiency** may cause irregular heart beat, nausea, weakness and mental derangements. **Food sources** are in all foods in varying amounts but are highest in legumes, nuts, whole grains and green vegetables. Too much magnesium can cause nausea, vomiting, lower blood pressure and heart problems. Excess amounts from food are unlikely to cause harm except in cases of kidney disease preventing magnesium from being excreted.

Chromium works with insulin to help the body use glucose and maintain proper blood sugar. **Deficiency** may cause symptoms resembling diabetes, such as impaired glucose tolerance and nerve damage. **Food sources** include meat, whole grains and nuts. The effects of too much chromium are not fully understood and are being studied.

Copper is essential in making hemoglobin, which carries oxygen in the blood. It is also an essential part of many body enzymes helping the body cells produce their needed energy. **Deficiency** is rare, except from certain genetic problems or by consuming too much zinc, which can hinder copper absorption. **Food sources** are organ meats, especially liver, seafood, nuts and seeds. Too much copper can cause nausea, vomiting, diarrhea, coma and liver damage, but is rare.

Fluoride helps harden tooth enamel, protecting teeth from decay. It may also help protect against osteoporosis by strengthening bones. **Deficiency** causes weak tooth enamel and may promote decay. **Food sources** may include tea especially if made with fluoridated water and fish with edible bones, such as canned salmon. Many communities add fluoride to the water supply, and fluoride supplements may be used with a doctor's supervision. Toothpaste is often made with fluoride enrichment. Too much fluoride can mottle or stain otherwise healthy teeth. It can also lead to brittle bones, increasing the frequency of bone fractures.

Iodine is an important part of thyroxin or thyroid hormone, which regulates the body's rate of energy use. **Deficiency** will interfere with thyroxin production, slowing the rate at which the body burns energy. Symptoms include weight gain, goiter and hypothyroidism. Because of the use of iodized salt in the United States and other parts of the world we have virtually eliminated iodine deficiency as a cause of goiter in the in most of the developed countries of the world. **Food sources** include saltwater fish and foods grown near coastal areas. Iodine is added to salt. Ironically, too much iodine may also cause goiter, but rarely at levels consumed in the United States.

Iron is an essential part of hemoglobin, which carries oxygen to body cells. **Deficiency** causes anemia, fatigue and infections. Deficiencies are more common among women with heavy menstrual periods. **Food sources** from animals are better absorbed than plant sources. These sources include meat, poultry, seafood, legumes, nuts and seeds, breads, cereals and other grain products. **Supplementation can be dangerous.** Adult iron supplements can be harmful to children; seek immediate medical attention if children accidentally take adult iron supplements. Iron supplements should also not be taken by men, post menopausal women without medical supervision. People with a genetic problem called hemochromatosis should not take iron supplements.

Water - Too often, we neglect the importance of proper hydration. Our nutrition must provide sufficient water required as a solvent, a transport medium, a substrate in hydrolytic reactions and for lubrication. Water makes up about 70% of our total body weight. Water needs continual replacement as it is lost from our bodies in urine, sweat, evaporation from lungs and in excrement. An average person requires 2-4 quarts of water a day supplied through drinks and liquid in our foods. Even a deficit of about 20% of our water needs can cause serious dysfunctions in our physical and mental abilities.

The idea is that once you discover how to detect foods that are unhealthy for you and your family, you'll avoid them. Don't let them be easily available for frequent consumption. Don't let them back into your home except on very special and rare occasions. Don't let them back into your habit system. Let them only be a rare treat—or better yet find a healthier treat to take their place. And above all don't use the kids as an excuse! It amazes us how often parents will say, "I know I shouldn't eat this, but I keep it in the house for the kids."

If it's unhealthy for you it's unhealthy for the kids! DON'T TEACH THEM YOUR BAD HABITS!

CHAPTER 6

ALL THAT NUTRITIONAL JARGON SIMPLIFIED...

You needn't be a nutritionist to successfully develop nutritionally sound eating habits for yourself, but the more you know about the language of nutrition the easier it will be to understand the fundamentals of healthy eating. That is really what we are talking about here—*healthy eating habits vs. unhealthy eating habits*. If you have healthy eating habits you need never again worry about that ugly buzz word "d--t!"

The better you understand the language of nutrition, the better equipped you'll be to shop properly and defensively. There is a lot of deception in the labeling of foods because much of the language of nutrition has been created by Madison Avenue and the marketing people of the food industry. Words such as "natural," "organic," "low sugar," "salt free," "lite," "low sodium," "no cholesterol," on the labels can be deceptive and confusing and more often than not, on purpose.

A big part of understanding nutrition is learning its special vocabulary. Let's take a look at the meaning of this special terminology of nutrition and thus arm ourselves to make wise decisions about our eating habits.

THE VOCABULARY OF NUTRITION

Absorption - the process of transforming nutrients and water from the stomach or intestinal track through the walls of the digestive system into the blood after digestion.

Amino acids - Organic compounds made up of the elements carbon, hydrogen, oxygen, nitrogen and in some cases sulfur. Amino acids are the building blocks of proteins.

Additives - chemicals added to food to enhance appearance, taste, texture, and in some cases nutritional value. Preservatives are the most common additives used to retard spoilage and prevent growth of disease causing micro-organisms.

Ascorbic acid - vitamin C.

Biochemistry - the chemistry of animals, plants or of all living things.

Bioflavonoid - a substance found mainly in the pulp of citrus fruits and once named vitamin P. Its nutritional value or need is doubtful in the minds of most authorities. Health food manufacturers often hype this as beneficial.

Biotin - one of the B complex vitamins. It is widely distributed in foods and is rarely deficient in humans.

Bran - is the tough, course and indigestible fiber coat of grains. Since it is not absorbed into the body it has no nutritional value but is a fiber and thus, extremely important to health for its mechanical role in digestion and elimination of harmful byproducts of digestion and biological functions.

Brewer's yeast - is a high-quality protein source rich in vitamins, phosphorus and iron.

Bulgur - cracked wheat retaining its bran, germ and nutrients.

Caffeine - a chemical compound found naturally in many foods such as coffee, tea and colas, which has a stimulating property to many people.

Calcium - an elemental mineral which is essential to bone structure, blood clotting, muscle tone, proper nerve transmission and other biologic functions.

Calorie - a unit by which heat is measured; the amount of heat required to raise the temperature of one gram of water one degree centigrade. It thus becomes a valuable measure of the energy source value of food. If a person consumes more calories than are needed to provide the energy demands of his/her lifestyle, the excess calories are converted to fat for storage.

Carbohydrate - a group of organic substances containing carbon, hydrogen, oxygen and designated as simple or complex. Simple carbohydrates are sugars; complex carbohydrates are the starches. Both are essential nutrients found abundantly in grains, fruits, starchy vegetables and milk. One gram of carbohydrate will produce four calories of energy.

Carbon - a chemical element present in all organic substances or substances derived from living organisms. Compounds not containing carbon are classified as inorganic or derived from non-living sources.

Carcinogen - a substance capable of causing cancer.

Carotene - a carbon, hydrogen compound that occurs in many vegetables and is a form of vitamin A that has cancer retarding properties as an anti-oxidant.

Catalyst - a substance that speeds or enhances chemical reactions, as in digestion, but is itself not used in the reaction; enzymes are catalysts.

Cell - the minimal, microscopic, functional structure of animal or plant life.

Chemical additives - synthetically compounded substances added to processed foods to enhance their flavor, color, texture or preservation.

Cholesterol - a constituent of animal fat which is produced in the body, mainly by the liver and is essential to many body processes and life itself. The body is capable of producing all the cholesterol it needs so heavy ingestion of dietary cholesterol in animal fats can lead to excessive deposition of cholesterol into the walls of blood vessels creating potential circulatory blockage. The greatest danger of these fat or atherosclerotic deposits is their potential contribution to heart attack and stroke. Excessive cholesterol has also been related to certain cancers. Cholesterol can be divided into high and low density lipids, HDL or LDL cholesterol. HDL is also known as "good cholesterol" while LDL is "bad cholesterol." HDL tends to protect the body from LDL when it is present in sufficient quantity. Thus it is important to have a low ratio of LDL to HDL. This ratio is more important than the cholesterol count itself.

Cruciferous vegetables - are members of the cabbage family, high fiber and potentially protective against certain cancers; kale, cauliflower, broccoli and Brussels sprouts.

Culture - microorganisms such as yeasts, molds and bacteria used to produce cheeses, fermented foods and drinks, buttermilk and breads.

Curd - the semisolid formed when milk is exposed to acid or certain enzymes; the semisolid part of cottage cheese.

Dietetics - the applied science of nutrition to the feeding of people.

Digestion - breaking down of food into its simple components in the digestive tract so that it can be absorbed into the body and utilized.

Endosperm - the starchy portion in a kernel of corn, wheat or other cereal grain, from which refined flour or meal is produced after the germ and outer fiber layers are removed.

Enzymes - are catalysts or substances that potentiate chemical reactions in the body without them entering into the reaction.

Factor - any chemical substance found in food, nutrient or non-nutrient.

Fat - an essential nutrient of plant or animal origin. Only about one tablespoon of unsaturated fat is needed daily for good nutrition. Fat supplies nine calories of energy per gram, making it more than twice as fattening as carbohydrate and protein when ingested in excess. Fats can be divided into "saturated" and "unsaturated." Saturated fats, most often derived from animal and dairy foods, are usually hard at room temperatures, like butter and lard. Saturated fats tend to raise the bad LDL cholesterol levels of the blood and are considered nutritionally unhealthy whether they come from animal or vegetable sources. Coconut oil and palm oil are vegetable fats that have properties similar to saturated animal fats, though they do not have cholesterol, they do tend to raise blood cholesterol when ingested. Unsaturated fats when hydrogenated take on the unhealthy characteristics of saturated fats. Unsaturated fats, polyunsaturated fats and monounsaturated fats are liquid at room temperatures (oils) and are usually vegetable in origin. They tend to lower bad LDL blood cholesterol while raising the good HDL cholesterol. Some vegetable fats have been treated chemically (hydrogenated) to solidify them at room temperature as in the case of margarine. This reduces their health benefits considerably. Monounsaturated fats (Canola oil and olive oil) tend to lower LDL and raise HDL. But they are still fats and should be used sparingly; however, when fat has to be used, these, Canola and Olive, are two you should utilize.

Fat-soluble - substances that won't dissolve in water but dissolve in fats and oils. Vitamins A, D, E and K are fat soluble.

Fiber - the indigestible substance in our foods, usually originating from plants. Fruits, vegetables and grains are all rich in fiber if it is not processed out. Most Americans consume about half the recommended fiber for good nutrition; about 30 grams is healthy. Eating more fiber controls digestion and elimination of waste and toxins from our bodies, helps reduce cholesterol absorption and decreases the risk of certain types of cancer.

Folic acid - one of the B complex vitamins essential in our nutrition. Deficiency will lead to anemia and blood disorders.

Fortified - food that has had nutrients added to make it more nutritionally valuable than in its original state. Milk is usually fortified with vitamin D which makes its natural calcium better absorbed and utilized by the body.

Fructose - levulose - fruit sugar. There is a misconception that fruit sugar is not as fattening as refined sugar or sucrose. Fruit sugar is about 70% sweeter than sucrose or table sugar, so you can get the same degree of sweetness with about 30% less calories, but fructose when eaten in excess has similar properties to table sugar.

Germ - the part of the grain which grows and allows plants to reproduce themselves. Germ is rich in vitamins and oils.

Glucose - dextrose - blood sugar - glucose is the body's main energy source. It is the main fuel for brain and muscle. Carbohydrates are the body's best source for glucose because they are easily converted into glucose. For this reason d--ts poor in carbohydrates are dangerous.

Gram - the basic unit of weight in the metric system. One ounce = 28.35 grams. One pound = 453.59 grams.

Honey - a sugar compound made up of fructose and a trace of glucose and a few trace minerals. It is sweeter than sucrose per calorie, but has no health benefits over table sugar. Though it requires a few less calories to get the same sweetening power, honey is more damaging to teeth and has been known to cause lethal botulism poisoning in infants.

Health foods - a very loose and overused term generally taken to include "naturally grown" or "organically grown" foods, as well as vegetarian foods, special dietary foods, foods specially high in nutritious value and foods produced free of chemicals and additives. All these poorly defined words, terms and phrases offer no guarantee that these "health foods" are any better for you. The only guarantee is that they are probably more expensive than the non-"health foods."

Hydrogenation - the addition of hydrogen to any unsaturated fat, usually a vegetable oil. Hydrogenation is the process by which oils are changed into solids, such as vegetable oils being changed into margarine.

Inorganic - chemical compounds which do not contain the element carbon and thus are not derived from once living material.

International Unit - I.U. - a measure of vitamin potency.

Lactose - milk sugar.

Lecithin - a fatty substance found in soybeans, corn, egg yolk and other plant and animal tissues with the property of being able to dissolve cholesterol deposits in one's body. Our bodies are capable of producing lecithin in varying amounts which may explain why some of us are more protected from high cholesterol than others.

Lipids - another term for fats, fat-like substances and oils.

Lyte/Lite - a marketing term that infers lower calories or fat in a product, but in no way guaranteeing this.

Macro biotics - a d--t based on whole grain foods.

Micro biotic - pertaining to microscopic plants or animals such as bacteria, molds and yeasts.

Minerals - inorganic substances, which like vitamins, their organic counterparts, are essential to life. Iron, potassium, calcium, zinc, iodine, copper, phosphorus, sodium and chloride are a few of the essential minerals we need for health and life maintenance.

Natural foods - a loosely defined term which usually means food produced with minimal processing, refining and no additives or produced with no chemical fertilizers, hormones, pesticides of antibiotics. The label "Natural," however, does not guarantee any of the above.

Nutrients - substances needed by the body for life and health which cannot be produced by the body itself and thus must be obtained from foods we eat.

Organic - those chemical compounds which contain carbon and which are obtained from living or once living matter.

Phytochemicals - these are plant chemicals that have protective or disease preventive properties and number more than thousand known phytochemicals to date. It is well-known that plants produce these chemicals to protect themselves and recent research indicates that they can protect humans against diseases too. Some of the well-known phytochemicals are lycopene found in tomatoes, isoflavones found in soy and flavanoids found in fruits. They are non-essential nutrients and are not required by the human body for sustaining life.

Protein - an essential nutrient made up of amino acids and necessary for tissue growth and repair. Protein derived from animal tissue is usually complete, containing all the essential amino acids. Plant protein is usually incomplete and must be eaten in combinations of vegetation to be as nutritional as animal protein.

Preservatives - chemicals that inhibit spoilage or growth of microorganisms. Preservatives are particularly important where proper refrigeration or freezing are not available.

P/S ratio - expresses the relative amount of unsaturated fat to saturated fat in oils or margarine. The higher the number, the higher the amount of unsaturated fat the product contains. Thus, the higher the P/S ratio number the healthier the product.

Riboflavin - vitamin B2 - one of the B complex vitamins.

Roughage - is another name for Fiber.

Salt - the common name given to sodium chloride or common table salt. Most Americans consume far more salt than is needed by the body, partly because of its excessive use in food processing. Excessive salt is associated with increased blood pressure in people at risk for hypertension.

Sodium - a mineral found in many foods and the inorganic element which forms common table salt when combined with chloride. It is sodium which causes hypertension when excess salt is ingested by those at risk for the disease. There are some studies at present that sodium in other forms than table salt are not as harmful in causing hypertension. A person should limit his or her sodium ingestion to less than 3000 mgs/day.

Starch - complex carbohydrate found in grains, potatoes, vegetables as opposed to the simple carbohydrates, i.e., sugars.

Sugar - simple carbohydrate as found in fruits and other plants. Sugars have very little nutritional value other than providing flavor and calories.

Transfats - transfats are neither required nor beneficial for health as are other fats. Transfats increases the risk of coronary artery disease and stroke. Health authorities worldwide recommend that consumption of transfat be reduced to bare minimums. Transfats from partially hydrogenated oils, saturated fats or unsaturated fats are generally considered to be far more of a health risk than fats occurring naturally.

Vitamins - organic substances derived from plants and animals which help to regulate metabolism and body functions. There are sixteen required vitamins each with several unique functions in life processes. The fat soluble vitamins A, D, E and K can be stored in body fat so they needn't be eaten on a daily basis. The water soluble vitamins C and B complex cannot be stored and must be included in our daily nutrition.

This glossary of basic terms is not intended to make you into a nutritionist, but it should help you to understand labels, advertisements and marketing ploys a little more to your advantage. More importantly, it should help you to understand better what might be harmful in your nutrition, what is good for you and what won't help or harm you. The basic idea of nutrition is to avoid what will harm you, seek out what is good for you... and enjoy or ignore the rest as you see fit. If you are interested in a deeper understanding of nutrition, which can only help you, we refer you to your local library which will have dozens of books on the topic. We also remind you to ignore the section of books on d--t and stick to the section on nutrition. There is a big difference between the two.

CHAPTER 7

IN DEFENSE OF FAT...

We're not here to tell you that fat is all good on you or for you. Far from it! But it isn't all bad either. God didn't put fat on us just to be mean or have a good laugh. Fat has a purpose and is essential to life.

We can see the purpose of fat a little easier when we look at its function on lower animals. Because of our adopted lifestyle, some of these needs and purposes for fat have become less obvious and important overtime. However, we still don't differ too much from animals in the wild.

Retention of heat...

Bears, otters, seals, whales and almost all other animals, including humans are insulated against cold weather by our sub-dermal layer of fat. Because of the garment industry this insulating layer of fat is not as important to us as it was to our cave dwelling ancestors. However, it can still be a lifesaving insulator under extreme conditions. It increases our survival time in cold water, extreme frigid weather or other forms of unexpected exposure. We heavier folks usually tolerate cold weather better because our bodies conserve heat better than our thinner friends.

Storage of energy...

Hibernating animals or animals that may be forced to fast for long periods of time between kills, rely upon their fat stores for energy. Because humans no longer depend on successful hunting, fat storage for long fasts is not often important, but as an energy source fat still plays a major role. The problem most of us have is that we deposit more storage fat than we burn off. Thus exercise is important to any weight or fat reduction or control program. Our bodies are marvels of efficiency and can get by on much less food energy than most of us tend to consume. The balance goes to fat storage deposits.

Raw materials for hormones and body functions...

If our bodies were devoid of fat, we could not produce hormones that are vital to life and reproduction. Additionally, there are fat soluble essential vitamins, body oils, enzymes, digestive fluids, brain and central nervous system tissues which rely on fats for their function, regeneration, production and maintenance.

Body contour...

Sub-dermal fat deposits when properly distributed give our bodies, especially female bodies, those desireable attractive curves that are so much desired. Sadly, these deposits are, all too often, not distributed the way we want them to be. Furthermore, this distribution is usually hereditary. Spot exercising which has been so popular to reshape the body, does not work for the majority of us. The idea is not to get rid of all the fat, but rather excess fat.

Floatation...

Fat is less dense than water thus weighing less, therefore it adds to buoyancy. This is of great importance to swimming animals, less important to us humans. In fact, when we scuba dive it becomes a problem and we have to wear a few pounds (actually more than a few pounds) of lead to help us get under.

Skin oils...

Oils are the liquid form of fat and thus, our body oils are fats. These are of great importance in maintaining a healthy skin and hair. Oils protect us from environmental assaults such as air, water, sun, heat and cold.

Trauma protection...

There are areas of fat around many of our vital organs which affords them protection from trauma. Just as Styrofoam packing insulates and protects precious and fragile objects from damaging impacts when shipped, so body fat reduces the chances of damage to delicate organs from blunt trauma.

These are but a few of the more important functions of body fat. A totally fat free d--t would be a serious detriment to our well being. Indeed, we could not long survive eating no fat. This does not mean I advocate total abandon when it comes to ingesting and storing fat. But it may be better for you to carry a little excess fat than to maintain a deficit in body fat. Fat is not all bad, as Madison Avenue would have you think. Some fats are very beneficial to our health!

Let's take a closer look at how much fat we should carry on our bodies and what kind of fats are safest for us to ingest. We don't want to eliminate fat from our nutrition, but rather exchange an acceptable quantity of healthy types of fats and oils in place of an unacceptable quantity of those fats and oils known to be detrimental to our health and longevity.

HEALTHY FATS AND OILS
vs.
THE BAD FATS AND OILS...

As a refresher to our memories, let's review our earlier definition of "fat:"

Fat - an essential nutrient of plant or animal origin. <u>Only about one tablespoon of unsaturated fat is needed daily for good nutrition.</u> Fat supplies nine calories of energy per gram, making it <u>twice as fattening as carbohydrate and protein</u> when ingested in excess. Fats can be divided into "saturated" and "unsaturated."

Saturated fats - usually derived from animal and dairy foods, are usually hard at room temperature, like butter and lard. Saturated fats tend to raise the bad LDL cholesterol levels of our blood and are to be considered nutritionally unhealthy. Coconut oil and palm oil are vegetable oils that have properties similar to saturated animal fats; though they do not have cholesterol, they do tend to raise the bad blood cholesterol (LDL) when ingested.

Unsaturated fats - monounsaturated and polyunsaturated are liquid at room temperatures (oils) and are usually vegetable in origin. They tend to lower blood bad LDL cholesterol and raise good HDL cholesterol. Fish oils are examples of oils derived from animals. Some vegetable fats have been treated chemically (hydrogenated) to solidify them at room temperature as in the case of margarine. Hydrogenation diminishes the health benefits of unsaturated fats.

Let me redirect you to a specific part of this definition:

"Fat - an <u>essential nutrient</u> of plant or animal origin. **Only about one tablespoon of unsaturated fat is needed daily for good nutrition. Fat supplies nine calories of energy per gram making it twice as fattening as carbohydrate and protein** when ingested in excess.

An average person requires about 15 Calories per day to maintain each pound of his/her body weight. That means a 150 pound person requires about 150 X 15 Calories, or 2250 Calories per day to maintain his/her weight. A 100 pounder would require 1500 daily Calories and a 200 pounder could eat 3000 Calories without altering his/her body weight. **A person should acquire less than 1/3 of those Calories from food fats according to the American Heart Association.** I personally feel you should try to hold that closer to 10% to 20% of your daily calories from fat, and those from monounsaturated fats which lower LDL and raise HDL.

"Fats" can be divided into saturated and unsaturated. Saturated fats, most often derived from animal and dairy foods, are usually hard at room temperatures, like butter and lard. Saturated fats tend to raise the cholesterol levels in our blood and are to be considered unhealthy. Coconut oil and palm oil are vegetable fats that have similar properties to saturated animal fats. They too should be avoided.

Othniel Seiden, MD & Jane L. Bilett, Ph.D.

COMPARISON OF DIETARY FATS IN ORDER OF THEIR HEALTHFULNESS

From the USDA Agricultural Handbook 8-4, 1979.

This table shows different dietary fats in decreasing order of healthfulness as to human use; Canola as healthiest and Coconut oil as least healthy. **Determination of healthfulness is how much the given fat or oil will tend to raise your blood cholesterol level.** You will notice that even though Palm Oil and Coconut Oil are vegetable fats and contain 0% cholesterol; their levels of saturated fat are so high they are less healthy for you than the listed animal fats. This shows you that just because a product boasts **"No Cholesterol!"** it is not necessarily good for you. You must learn to read labeled ingredients to get the whole story and avoid those products rich in saturated fats. Also, you must learn to limit your ingestion of the "good fats." Remember, the body needs only about two three teaspoons of fat per day; any more than that is excessive.

Unsaturated fats, polyunsaturated and monounsaturated are liquid at room temperature (oils) and are usually vegetable in origin. Fish oils are examples of oils derived from animals. **They tend to lower blood cholesterol.** Some vegetable oils have been treated chemically (hydrogenated) to solidify them at room temperature as in the case of margarine. **Hydrogenation diminishes the health benefits of unsaturated fats.**

HOW MUCH FAT IS RIGHT FOR YOU?

Fat does not necessarily cause death. Fat, however, is all too often a symptom of those factors that do cause untimely deaths. Too often, fat people are sedentary and a sedentary life-style tends to increase one's chances for an early death. If a person with some excess fat is also very active in aerobic activities he/she may well have a very healthy body capable of sustaining long life.

A fat person might be heavy because he/she eats too much of the wrong foods and therefore has a very high cholesterol with low HDL and high LDL. High cholesterol with low HDL and high LDL greatly increases one's chances for an early demise. On the other hand, a person might have a hereditary predisposition for being overweight even though he/she eats proper and nourishing foods maintaining a low total cholesterol with a relatively high HDL and low LDL. That person is not necessarily at higher risk of early death because of his higher body fat ratio.

Often folks who are under a great deal of stress tend to overeat as a defense mechanism. This can lead to excess fat deposits. The distress is the potential killer and the fat may only be a less lethal symptom of the distress. Another person who might be somewhat overweight with a little excessive fat to lean mass ratio, but who is not distressed, rather happy with his/her lot in life, may be at no great risk of early death or serious illness.

We are saying that excessive fat is a detriment to good health, but a moderate amount of body fat may well be better for you than trying constantly to attain an unrealistic weight goal.

So, how much fat is acceptable?

Let's consider body fat in terms of heart attack risk. The following table indicates heart attack risks as; very low, low, moderate, high and very high and correlates them with varying body fat percentages in men and women:

HEART ATTACK RISK FACTOR OF VARIOUS BODY FAT PERCENTAGES

Remember, these risks are affected by other factors. If you are under great stress, smoke, eat foods that are poor in nutrition, have high blood pressure, are diabetic, do not exercise regularly in a vigorous aerobic program and/or have a family history of heart disease, you may be pushed into a high risk category even though your body fat may only be in the low to moderate range.

Age also affects what is acceptable body fat percentages. As we get older, we can carry a little more fat and still consider ourselves fit—to a point. The following tables show how age affects permissible body fat percentages in various fitness categories among men and women:

EXCELLENT FITNESS & BODY FAT %
GOOD FITNESS & BODY FAT %
AVERAGE FITNESS & BODY FAT %
POOR FITNESS AND BODY FAT %
VERY POOR FITNESS AND BODY FAT %

You'll notice, nothing has been said about weight in these tables of fitness and body fat percentages. You could be lighter in weight than another person of your same height and bone structure and still have a higher body fat percentage than he/she or vice versa. You should notice that there is a range of percentages for each fitness category. This simply indicates that a person, who may have a little higher body fat ratio than another person, can still be more fit than that other person. You will also notice that nothing is mentioned about body fat percentages and health status. Body fat percentage is no guaranteed indicator of health status. There are thin people of relative poor health and relatively fat people of extremely good health around. True, a person in good fitness has a much better chance of being in good health, but not all thin people are fit and not all heavy folks are unfit.

What this all boils down to is that you must find your own ideal body weight and it will not be at a point on a weight chart, but rather somewhere near the best body fat percentage for your age and gender category.

That leads us to the tough question, "How does one determine one's body fat percentage?"

FINDING YOUR BODY FAT PERCENTAGE...

There are several ways to have your body fat percentage determined, but sad to say, none are as simple as stepping on a scale.

WATER IMMERSION METHOD...

This method of determining percentages of body fat requires weighing the subject out of water and then completely submerged in water. After obtaining your "dry" weight on a regular scale, usually dressed in a swim suit, you are seated on a submersible disk suspended from another scale. The disk is then lowered into a pool or tank with you on board and your submerged weight is recorded. The test

DIETARY FAT %	CHOLESTEROL %	SATURATED %	UNSATURATED SOURCE	
			%Poly	%Mono
Canola Oil	0%	6%	32%	62%
Olive Oil	0%	14%	9%	77%
Safflower Oil	0%	10%	77%	13%
Sunflower Oil	0%	11%	69%	20%
Corn Oil	0%	13%	62%	25%
Soybean Oil	0%	15%	61%	24%
Peanut Oil	0%	18%	33%	49%
Cottonseed Oil	0%	25%	50%	25%
Lard	12%	41%	12%	47%
Beef Tallow	14%	52%	4%	44%
Butter Fat	33%	66%	4%	30%
Palm Oil	0%	83%	2%	15%
Coconut Oil	0%	92%	2%	6%

depends on accurately determining the difference in your weight "on land" and "fully submerged" with as much air exhaled out of your lungs as you can possibly breathe out. Very fat people weigh much less under water than those who have little fat on them. The weight difference between dry and wet weight is plugged into a formula along with other of your measurements—and out comes your body fat percentage.

The problems with this test are several and obvious. It's

difficult to find a facility which has the equipment to do this weighing method. Some health clubs have the equipment, but usually it requires a major hospital or medical teaching center to find this test available. Additionally, it is a fairly expensive test to administer, $50 to $150. The test is highly accurate providing the person administering it knows what he/she is doing and makes sure you empty your lungs of air as completely as possible. The test's accuracy is very dependent on the cooperation of the person being tested and results from one operator to another can vary greatly.

CALIPER FAT FOLD
MEASUREMENT METHOD...

In this method, a pair of special calipers is utilized to pinch up a fold of fat on several locations of your body. The person measuring then gets an accurate index of the thickness of your subcutaneous fat in various parts of the body. These numbers are then applied to tables which have been established to be within 3% to 4% accurate over the years. Unlike the underwater weighing method, this test can be found in many doctor's offices, health clubs and spas, hospitals, and clinics. It is also much less costly and should never be over $15. Many clubs will do it as a courtesy for their members or prospective members. As with any test, it is only as good as the person administering it and if that person is inexperienced or lacking training, there could be a high percentage of error. If five different people administer this test on one individual, there is a fair chance they will come up with three to five different results. These results will, however be within a few percentage points of one another.

ELECTRIC RESISTANCE METHOD...

Also known as the **Bioelectrical Impedance Method**, it is accurate to within 3% to 5%, depending on your age and hydration. As you get older, the accuracy diminishes a little, and if it is carried out after a workout where you've perspired a lot, its accuracy might be diminished. It works on the principle that fat, muscle and other body tissues all conduct electric current with different resistance. A very mild and completely painless current is sent through you between electrodes attached to your body and a reading is given off by the calibrated electronic unit stating your percentage body fat. Many doctors, hospitals, clinics and health clubs have the equipment, and the cost for the test may run anywhere from gratis to $20. This method is probably the most consistently accurate measure of body fat percentage and has least dependence on administration experience. Any number of different operators should get the same result when testing any one individual.

INFRARED WAND METHOD...

The technical name of this method is **The Near-Infrared Interactance Method.** The equipment is not as readily available to the general public as the caliper or bioelectrical methods, but it is simple, quick and usually inexpensive. A wand which sends an infrared beam into the body is placed against a spot on the arm. It works on the principle that fatty tissue absorbs the infrared at a different rate than other tissue and thus it measures the thickness up subcutaneous fat. By formula, the device calculates the percentage of body fat and gives a reading. Because the method is calculated on only one area of the body, it is less accurate than other methods. Its cost should range from gratis to $25. As with the caliper and submersion methods, this method will depend somewhat on the expertise of the administrator.

We believe that body fat percentage determination will become far more common in the near future bringing down the cost of the procedure and greatly increasing the accuracy of the tests. We wouldn't even be surprised to see technology make an inexpensive accurate home testing procedure available in the near future.

Once you have determined what your body fat percentage is, you will have a choice to make. You can choose to bring it to a more acceptable level by increasing your muscle mass or by lowering your fat. More than likely you will choose a combination of the two. **When you attain a percentage of** body fat in a fitness area that you feel your best, you will probably be very near your own ideal body weight. That is a primary goal of this program.

But since we are not going to use weight as a major method of evaluating your progress and fitness, we need other criteria or surveying our improvement. To achieve this, let's move on to the next step which should help you to set new and realistic goals for yourself—Weights and Measures...

	Very Low	Low	Moderate	High	Very High
Women	15%	20%	25%	33%	40%>
Men	12%	16%	22%	25%	30%>

CHAPTER 8

Age	20-29	30-39	40-49	50-59	60>
Men	7%-12%	7%-14%	9%-15%	9%-16%	10%-16%
Women	5%-12%	5%-14%	7%-16%	10%-18%	7%-18%

Age	20-29	30-39	40-49	50-59	60>
Men	14%-16%	16%-18%	17%-19%	18%-20%	17%-19%
Women	15%-18%	16%-19%	19%-20%	22%-25%	22%-25%

Age	20-29	30-39	40-49	50-59	60>
Men	18%-22%	20%-22%	21%-24%	22%-25%	20%-24%
Women	22%-26%	22%-26%	23%-27%	27%-30%	27%-30%

Age	20-29	30-39	40-49	50-59	60>
Men	25%-28%	25%-28%	26%-28%	27%-29%	27%-29%
Women	27%-31%	27%-31%	29%-31%	32%-33%	31%-33%

Age	20-29	30-39	40-49	50-59	60>
Men	29%>	29%>	30%>	30%>	33%>
Women	35%>	35%>	35%>	35%>	35%>

WEIGHTS AND

MEASURES....

If you're sick of stepping up on the scale and being frustrated with what you see, then this chapter is for you! Every d--t book you pick up is based on your losing pounds and pounds and more pounds. When you go to a physician and he or she puts you on a d--t, your physician will probably follow your progress, success or failure, completely by weight change.

There are a number of measures and indexes of your health status that are far better indicators than what you tip your scale to. We have been misled to believe that if you don't look like a model or match a number on a weight chart that we are unacceptable and in terrible health. Let's look at these other measures that are better indexes of your health status.

YOUR IDEAL BODY WEIGHT....

We've mentioned this concept before; let's reexamine it a bit closer. Two people might be the same height and have the same bone structure. One might be of average stature, slim and right on the button with his weight as the weight chart recommends. The second fellow may be very athletic, well muscled, broad shouldered with full biceps and triceps, heavily muscled thighs and calves and a hard flat stomach. Because of his well muscled body, he wears a coat two sizes larger than his slimmer counterpart. He may also wear a belt two inches smaller than the scrawny man because of his well toned and flat abdomen. Because muscle tissue is relatively heavy compared to fatty tissue, our athletic friend may outweigh his more sedentary counterpart by twenty or thirty pounds or more. According to the weight chart the more athletic person is "overweight," and by its standards, "unfit!" Our other friend, the less athletic more sedentary of the two, is right on with the weight chart, inferring that he is more "fit," healthier, right where he should be to live a long healthy life. Right?

Wrong!

Our athletic, well muscled friend, though thirty or more pounds heavier probably has far less body fat than his sedentary friend, in actual fat mass and percentage body fat. And since the lighter of the two is sedentary, he has less energy, less endurance, less strength, less resistance to illness, less resistance to injury and worst of all he has a far worse cardiovascular and cardiopulmonary status. Chances are the thinner of our two friends has a higher blood pressure and a much higher pulse rate at rest and during exertion. Blood analysis will probably show his cholesterol to be higher with a low HDL (good cholesterol) and high LDL (bad cholesterol) when compared to his heavier counterpart. Ironically the thinner of the two will have an easier time buying life and health insurance. Insurance companies like people to fit the charts.

The fact remains though, our heavier friend is much closer, if not right on his Ideal Body Weight and our thinner friend might be right on the weight chart but under his Ideal Body Weight.

Bill's heavy friend, call him Jack, convinces his thin but sedentary buddy, Bill, that he should get more active. They go to work out together. Bill isn't interested in building a muscular body like Jack's, but wants to firm up and strengthen his heart, lungs, circulatory system to develop more endurance.

Bill, being right on the spot as far as his weight chart states, does not feel he needs to d--t, but Jack shows him that he could eat more healthier foods. If he'd watch his fat and sugar consumption closer and add high fiber foods to his daily consumption. Nothing was said about the quantity of food he should eat, only the quality. Calories aren't discussed. Jack also gets Bill to join him in his daily <u>aerobic</u> workout. Since Bill isn't interested in building a more muscular body, Jack doesn't involve him in his anaerobic body building workouts which he does three times a week in addition to his aerobics.

Over the next few weeks Bill has some surprises:

1. Weight gain
2. Clothes get loose
3. Increased energy
4. Pulse slows
5. Blood pressure falls
6. Muscles tone up
7. Distress reduces
8. Production increases
9. Feels better
10. Confidence grows
11. Others comment positively
12. Enjoys life a lot more

WEIGHT GAIN....

Bill's biggest surprise was an initial weight gain. After all, he was watching his nutritional intake closer and though he wasn't on a d--t, he'd made every effort to reduce his fat consumption and had markedly increased his fiber intake. Why wouldn't that make him lose weight, especially since he was vigorously engaging in an aerobic exercise program?

The answer is simple!

Fat weighs less than muscle!

The reduction of fat and increased fiber consumption began to melt away the body fat Bill did have, though there never was much there, and the calories he burned in his aerobic exercise helped to burn it off too. But the exercise did something more. It began to tone his muscles and actually put some muscle mass on his bones, especially in his legs, back, stomach and shoulders. The net result was a slight weight gain. He left his perfect perch on the weight chart and gained toward his own Ideal Body Weight. His percentage of body fat was reducing, muscle mass was increasing and he actually gained weight, <u>but it was healthy weight.</u>

Had Bill just been following his weight as it pertained to a weight chart, as most people and physicians do when starting on a d--t, he would have considered his program a failure and detrimental to his health status. Thus he realized that weight was the least important of measures that determine his physical conditioning. Bill began taking greater interest in other signs and measures of his successful progress.

CLOTHING BEGAN TO FIT LOOSE...

In spite of his slight weight gain, Bill began to notice that his clothing began to fit him loose in places. It began to make sense that, if fat weighed less than muscle, a pound of fat would take up more space than a pound of muscle. Thus, if he exchanged a pound of fat for a pound of muscle, his body mass would actually diminish just because there would be less total tissue there.

Furthermore, by toning his muscles there was less sagging. Though weight went on, inches around the belt came off. A toned stomach takes up less space than a sagging belly.

A simple tape measure could tell him more than his expensive new electronic state-of-the-art scale. He began taking weekly measurements around his waist, hips, chest, thighs and neck.

INCREASED ENERGY...

Activity breeds on activity. As the percentage of body fat comes down and the muscle and muscle tone increase, strength increases. Excess baggage diminishes.

Cardiovascular and cardiopulmonary efficiency increased and energy abounded. Most importantly, the desire to be sedentary began to fade. A healthy body wants to be active. As his energy increased, Bill wanted more activity.

PULSE SLOWS....

As the heart becomes stronger through aerobic exercise, it also becomes more efficient. Its stroke volume increases; more blood is pumped with each contraction. More oxygen gets to the muscles and organs of the body with less effort on the part of the heart. As a result, Bill's resting pulse went down because his now healthier heart doesn't have to beat as often to supply his resting body with oxygen and blood supply to keep it functioning. By the same token, his heart doesn't have to work

> It is the premise of this program
> that weight is the least important
> measure of your success
> at turning your health status around.

as hard during activity to keep him going. The exercise that raised his pulse to 150 beats/minute when he first started working out, now only raises it to 140 beats/minute. To get the same cardiopulmonary benefit Bill has to increase his activity rate to bring his pulse back up to 150 and so his exercise pulse rate continues to determine how hard he works out.

BLOOD PRESSURE FALLS....

One of the best methods of bringing down blood pressure is to exercise. A one hour a day, vigorous aerobic exercise program will do more to bring an elevated blood pressure down for most people than all the medications in the world. Reducing blood pressure is one of the best measures of your general fitness. As you approach your Ideal Body Weight, your blood pressure should also approach an ideal level for you.

MUSCLES TONE UP....

If your exercise program tends to raise your weight slightly, don't look for increased fat deposits to account for it. Chances are you're putting on some new muscle tissue. See if your flab isn't being replaced by stronger well-toned muscle. Your belt might move in a few notches and that means more than the change on your scale, regardless which way it may go. Your clothes might get a little tight in the chest and thighs and looser in the waist and hips. These are far better signs than your relative position on a weight chart.

DISTRESS REDUCES...

There is stress and distress. Stress is an important part of life. It is a motivator. It keeps us out of ruts. It makes us get up and do things. Stress is what made you get involved with this program. Something about your physical condition made you feel uneasy (stressed) enough to seek a solution to your less than satisfactory health status. Stress is good because it makes you dissatisfied with the status quo.

If on the other hand, you do nothing about your

dissatisfaction, or if you try to make changes and fail, stress becomes distress—and distress is not good. Distress leads to those life pressures and angers detrimental to your health. It is not stress that brings on heart attacks but the resultant state of unresolved anger when your stress motivated actions don't improve the stressing situation.

As your physical status improves you will notice a reduction in your distress and anger levels. Two factors contribute to this:

1. Exercise is one of the best reducers of distress and anger known to man. Exercise offers you an opportunity to "work off" hostility. Hostility reduction = anger reduction = lowered distress.

2. As your health status improves, you tend to attack your distressing problems with an energy and vigor that helps solve them before they have a chance to affect your health. When you notice things just don't get to you the way they used to, you can be sure you're making real progress. It beats anything your scales can tell you about yourself! Also, exercise stimulates right brain activity which helps to solve problems on a more subconscious level. Many times you'll start a workout with a quandary and when you finish your exercise you'll have a sudden revelation of a solution, not even realizing your right brain was actively solving your dilemma.

PRODUCTION INCREASES....

As your health status improves and your energy levels rise and things don't bother you as much as they did because they seem to get solved, your production level will rise dramatically. You'll get things done and go looking for more. Sitting on a couch watching TV just won't cut it for you anymore. You'll seek out new interests and activities. You'll find fun in things that were chores before and you'll find more time for the things you used to enjoy but for which you never seemed to have the energy or the time. When you begin to notice that new fullness and fulfillment in your life you can begin to worry less about what your scales say.

FEEL TERRIFIC....

Think about the way you've been feeling over the past few years. Try to remember what it's been like up to now, because as you get into your new lifestyle and health program you'll be amazed at how great you can feel when your health status turns around. Your new energy levels, endurance, interests, will let you know in no uncertain terms that you are getting better every day. Even if your weight stays the same or goes up a little, you'll know

> Bill realized that it made more sense
> to measure body circumferences
> once a week than to weigh
> body mass daily.

you're better off because you feel markedly better when your health is improving.

CONFIDENCE GROWS...

When everything is getting better, you'll notice there's a new confidence about you in everything you attempt. As you begin to solve your problems, have new energy to accomplish what you want, feel better each day, begin to take on a better shape, you can't help but develop a new found confidence in anything you want to do. Success begets success in everything you do.

OTHERS COMMENT...

Not only will you notice all the above mentioned changes in yourself, others will notice too. You'll start to hear comments like, "You look like you're losing weight!" (even if you aren't); or, "What's different about you?"; "You're a new man/woman!"; "You seem to have taken ten years off!"; or, "I can't get over the changes in you!" Those comments have to make you feel better than the comments you've probably been hearing for the last few years about yourself.

ENJOY LIFE...

When life becomes more and more of a joy each day, you don't have to get on a scale to know you're improving your health status. When was the last time you couldn't wait for morning to come so you could embrace life with a new-found vitality? That's what you should be looking forward to; not how much you gained or lost since yesterday.

Now if you want to weigh yourself for old time's sake, go ahead. Just remember what you see on the scale has little to do with how you are or how you feel!

CHAPTER 9

CLEAN UP YOUR ACT! STOP POISONING YOURSELF... & OTHERS...

The people in developing countries where long life and seeming immunity to heart disease and cancer is enjoyed <u>don't poison themselves!</u> We, on the other hand, seem to have an illogical love of deadly chemicals. If there is a chemical substance that destroys human tissue, we seem to seek it out to swallow it, sniff it, inhale it, inject it, smear it on ourselves or abuse ourselves with it in one way or another! Why?

Our greed and avarice makes us pollute our air and water supplies. In our headlong dash to escape realities and responsibilities, we contaminate our bloodstreams with tranquilizers, alcohol and illicit drugs. And in our desire to be "Virginia Slim" or "Macho Man," we let Madison Avenue and the tobacco industry seduce us into tobacco addiction.

It will take some time and legislation to clean up our environment, but we are heading in that direction, thanks to some fine organizations dedicated to restoring our planet to its preindustrial cleanliness. But we can't leave it to others. We must put pressure on our legislators, local and national, to act quickly and strongly with protective laws. Let them know you won't vote for them if they don't protect their constituents from industry's garbage. And let industries know you won't buy their products if they aren't responsible with their refuse and deadly by-products.

As for excessive and irresponsible use of alcohol, tranquilizers and illegal drugs, that's something you have to

> **A slowing pulse rate is one of the best indicators of cardiovascular/cardiopulmonary improvement.**

take responsibility for. First you have to recognize and admit you have a drug problem—an addiction. And then you have to get help. If you are dependent on the use of alcohol, tranquilizers, tobacco or illegal drugs then you have an addiction and you have to beat that addiction before you can turn your life and health around. To do this you must get help! Talk to your physician, your family, friends, clergy—to anyone who can give you support and direction in getting qualified counseling for your problem.

Of all the chemical substances and pollutants that are harmful to your health, none are more deadly than tobacco.

And if you, yourself, do not smoke, but live with, or work among smokers, they are drastically shortening your life and destroying your good health.

There is no chemical abuse more harmful to your health, heart and lungs than the 4000 poisons found in tobacco! Let me repeat that; no chemical abuse is more harmful to your cardiopulmonary or cardiovascular systems and your general health than tobacco products and the smoke they produce!

It matters not whether you smoke a pipe, cigars, cigarettes, chew or sniff. Tobacco is tobacco is tobacco! Low tars, high tars, filtered—it doesn't matter, tobacco is deadly poison to just about every tissue in your body and especially to your heart. Stop exposing yourself to tobacco products right now! Not tomorrow, or next week—**Quit Smoking Now!**

If you are not a smoker but live with a smoker or work with smokers that expose you to their side stream smoke, then give the Quit Smoking Now! program, found in the appendix of this book to the smoker (s) in your life. Your exposure to their smoke is deadly to you and will prevent you from making a full potential turn around in your health and lifestyle change. If they refuse to quit smoking then make them understand, **they must not smoke in your home and in your presence.** If you work among smokers make them understand that they have every right to injure themselves but they must not pollute the same air that non-smokers have to breathe.

Perhaps you think these are strong demands, but you cannot afford to take the chance of breathing second hand or side stream smoke anymore than you can continue smoking if indeed you are a smoker. What you must realize—and what you must make others realize—is that **side stream smoke, the smoke that comes off of the lit end of the cigarette, cigar or pipe while smoldering, is far more toxic, dangerous and deadly than the mainstream smoke the smoker inhales and blows out!**

When a smoker sucks on his cigarette, cigar or pipe, he/she pulls a tremendous current of fresh air through the lit tobacco tip. This rush of air with its supply of oxygen causes the tobacco to glow red and pushes the temperature of the lit tobacco up from the smoldering 250 degrees to a glowing 1200 degrees Fahrenheit temperature. At 1200 degrees, the tobacco burns far more efficiently than at a smoldering 250 degrees.

At 1200 degrees, much more of the 4,000 lethal chemicals found in tobacco are destroyed by burning them up. Thus, side stream smoke from the smoldering tobacco puts many times the lethal chemicals and tars into the air around the smoker for the non-smokers and the smokers to share. The smoker, of course, gets both the mainstream smoke and the side stream smoke.

Side stream smoke is a serious health hazard. It is estimated that side stream smoke shortens the lives of as many as 50,000 non-smokers a year. Most susceptible to the dangers of side stream smoke are children, the elderly and anyone who has a heart problem.

Let me repeat, if you are a smoker, Quit Smoking Now!— before you take your next cigarette, cigar or pipe. To help you, use the Quit Smoking Now! program in the appendix of this book. If you are a non-smoker, but live and work with smokers, make them understand that they must not smoke in the air that you and other non-smokers are forced to breathe!

Next to smoking, the greatest addiction in this country and the world is the addiction to alcohol. When it comes to alcohol we get mixed messages. There are those who will tell you, "a drink will benefit you by relaxing you and getting rid of your distress!" One drink, and not a very strong one at that, may relax you a bit, may help dilate your blood vessels a bit and may help you to digest your next meal a bit. By the same token, a strong drink, a second, third or more drinks will work as a depressant, constrict your blood vessels and cause severe gastric irritation and retard digestion. If you can limit yourself to a glass of wine or beer after work or before dinner, booze probably won't hurt you and indeed might do you a bit of good. However, if you're the person who can't stop with just one, two at the most, you might have a drinking problem— and if you have a drinking problem you have to stay away from alcohol completely!

Alcohol addiction affects about one in five of our

population. It cuts across all social, economic, racial, professional, educational and age levels. It is equally distributed among the sexes. If drinking has caused you problems in the past, now is the time to get help. Your life depends on getting help!

Even if you do not have a problem with alcohol, moderate consumption can be dangerous if you are on medication. The blood thinner Coumarin, for example, is very much affected by alcohol consumption and may be thrown out of control by occasional "partying." Be sure you discuss your drinking habits honestly with your physician if you are on any medication at all. And if you find you can't discuss your drinking honestly with others, you have a drinking problem!

One area of drug abuse that all too often is overlooked is the misuse of prescription drugs. It is not uncommon anymore, especially among the elderly, to become addicted to medications prescribed originally for justifiable reasons. Again, it is essential that you review all your medications routinely with your physician. This is especially true if you see more than one doctor for your overall health care. Too frequently one medical advisor does not know what another is prescribing and you could be taking medications that either counteract each other, potentiate each other or cause one or the other to react differently than is intended.

It is also wise to get all your prescriptions and medications at one pharmacy so that the pharmacist can monitor what you are taking and see the overall picture of your medical regimen. Your pharmacist can be your greatest ally when it comes to keeping you safe from prescription misuse and abuse.

Of course, if you use illegal drugs you must get professional help. Here again, denial is the biggest problem. Let me make one flat statement: "There is no such thing as casual or recreational illicit drug use!" If you use illicit drugs only occasionally, you are a person in need of help. You are a time bomb waiting to go off! Your habit will get stronger and worse—it is just a matter of time—and not a lot of time at that. Get help now to kick the habit or deteriorate physically, mentally, economically, socially to your ultimate death! Get help now!

Hopefully, you are among the majority of our population who are not afflicted by chemical abuses. If so consider yourself lucky and go on to the next chapter in this program. If you are addicted to any one or more of the abused chemicals, recognize that this is another illness that you have to deal with and get help today!

CHAPTER 10

YOUR LIFE MAY DEPEND ON YOUR ATTITUDE...

Stress and Distress—REPRIORITIZE....

If there is one remarkable similarity among the primitive folks in those high longevity areas of the world we've been

> **If you use any tobacco product you are drastically shortening your life!**

mentioning, it's the lack of *distress* and more important, *anger*, in their lives. I make a point to emphasize the word "distress." Much has been written about stress and stress reduction in past years. But stress is not the problem. Distress and its resultant *anger* is what *kills* us Americans.

Stress is normal to life. It is what motivates us to get things done. It pushes us off dead center. Makes us climb out of ruts. It's when we can't do anything about the stress that we get distressed and angry. It is the distress and anger and their accompanying frustrations, irritations, feelings of futility, failure and disappointment causing even deeper anger that destroy out health and shorten our lives.

For most of us "distress and anger" are the most difficult aspects of our lifestyles to eliminate or change. Too many of us have set goals that are too demanding, unrealistic or plain impossible for ourselves. For some crazy reason, we insist on "keeping up with Jones," or worse, "we want to be the Jones!"

Fortunately, as we get older, most of us tend to mellow out a bit and distress and anger become less of a factor in our lives. Furthermore, when life threatening illness comes along, it seems to help us put aside some of the crazy goals that have caused us so much distress in our lives. Brushes with severe illness and crises tend to help us REPRIORITIZE our lives and values. Hopefully, this chapter will help you to do just that; REPRIORITIZE your life and values <u>before they cause the distress and anger</u> that bring on life threatening illnesses and crises. You must learn to let distress and anger play a very minimal role during your long, active and healthy, happy future.

What can we learn about avoidance of distress and anger from our primitive friends?

Let's take a look at what material things they have in comparison to us. To begin with, in each of the geographic areas we've discussed, the people have adequate food to nourish themselves. Nature has provided well for them. They eat properly and they have plenty. They don't have a problem clothing themselves. They don't dress fancy but they keep warm and comfortable. They dress for the prevailing climate. In places where it gets cold, they add a few layers and wrap up in blankets; and where and when it's warm or hot, they strip down to the bare essentials. Patches don't bother them except in their "Sunday go to church" clothes.

They have a roof over their heads. The roof may shelter a whole extended family of a dozen or more in two or three rooms, but they stay dry when it rains, warm when it snows and shaded when the sun burns down. There's rarely a lock on the door, but because they don't have much there's little to steal. They don't have much, but they don't <u>crave</u> much. What is important to them are the necessities, the food on their table, the clothes on their back, the roof over their heads and the love and support of their extended family.

Now compare! Most of us have too much food on our tables. Our homes are much more than adequate. Our clothing is usually abundantly hung in closets and we are able to communicate with loved ones though not in the same house always. So if we're so much better off, why are we so "distressed and angry?"

Perhaps it's those *"cravings!"*

Now I'm certainly not suggesting we give up all our material and modern conveniences. Far from it. I have nothing against the "good life." But let's reexamine and make sure what we "crave" is really "good." Let's make sure the price we pay with "distress" isn't too high.

For example, in our society, most of us need a car. Our pace and distances are too great for us to rely on walking from appointment to appointment. We can buy a car for around $9,000 that will usually get us where we want to go with reasonable reliability and comfort. We can buy a $90,000 car and it will usually get us there with reasonable reliability and comfort—considerable more comfort—but probably not $81,000 more comfort. Ah, but the prestige; that may be worth $81,000 to some of us. If we can afford it, the luxury car may be a source of joy and happiness. That's where the "good life" may indeed be "good" for you.

But, if putting out that extra 81 grand causes too much sacrifice, hardship, sleeplessness, and a heap of "distress," that "good life" isn't good for you. It just can't be worth it. If it harms your health, rethink your priorities and values. Set a more realistic goal. Find another more affordable way to derive that prestige. I'd love to be able to drive a Rolls Royce

Silver Shadow Convertible, but I know the worry would kill me. Instead I bought a used 1970 Buick Skylark Convertible for under $2000. By the time I got it all restored I had less than $5000 tied up in it. It's a thrill to drive, lets me be a bit of a show off, makes me feel like I'm the envy of all those other folks in small, closed, new plastic cars. I get my prestige and kicks for about $140,000 less, even if it is a little shy of being a Silver Shadow.

Now is the best time for you to really REPRIORITIZE your life. Take a realistic inventory of your values. Is being at the top of your profession as important to you now as it once might have been? Is being the richest guy in the hospital or cemetery really what you want out of life? Are you going to be able to enjoy all you material possessions, or would you be better off with a few less "things" and a lot more "time" to enjoy your life and family, friends and loved ones?"

STRESS vs. DISTRESS

Stress as I used it in this book means a physical or mental tension, an uneasiness, an irritation, a pull, tug or force to bring about a change in the status quo. It does not infer pain, grief, suffering, strain, frustration. These characteristics I delegate to "distress."

I use stress as that good restlessness that provokes you to some action. Distress, on the other hand, is worry, frustration agony, pain, etc., resulting when your actions don't work out as desired. That brings on "anger" and anger is what will do you in. Anger is what will cause you hypertension, ulcers, heart attacks, strokes and a host of other dread diseases.

If you were a world class sprinter and had a shot at the Olympics, no doubt you would come under considerable stress prior to the tryouts. If that stress made you work out harder, resulting in top fitness, improving your chances, it would be good. If you felt no stress prior to the tryouts you probably wouldn't push yourself to attain peak conditioning. On the day of the tryouts you would probably feel the greatest stress and that would get your adrenalin flowing and add considerably to your chances of success. After the race, you would be elated and happy if you placed. All that stress of the previous weeks and months would have benefited you.

If on the other hand, you lost—didn't place, there would probably be considerable frustration, pain, "the agony of defeat,"—*distress* and its accompanying *anger!* If you didn't have a mechanism to cope with your distress and anger, it could lead to depression, anxiety, feelings of failure and eventually any number of physical and mental ailments.

Stresses remain beneficial as long as they provoke positive action. Once you let them turn to negative action or inaction or become worrisome and self-depreciating, you've got distress. If the loser of the Olympic trials turns his failure to make the team into positive action, he will be coping with his distress, turning it back into positive stress. He might decide to work harder and improve his performance, lest one of the winners would drop out and he be elected to the team as an alternate. Perhaps he might decide the event wasn't for him and turn his energies to another event such as team relay. He might decide he was finished with competition, that it was fun while it lasted and now it was time to turn to other goals. All these would be positive reactions to potential distress, defusing it by turning it into other motivating stresses. *The way to cope with distress is to "turn your lemons into lemonade!"*

When you have a setback, don't fret and stew about it. That does no good. Turn your energies into another direction and if need be, return to your problem at a later time when you can face it objectively.

Exercise is one of the best ways to defuse distress; and you may be surprised at how often a solution to your distress will come to you spontaneously while your attention is diverted to more pleasant activities.

If your life is constantly filled with distress and anger, it is time to take a full accounting of your situation. This may require the help of an objective outsider. Not necessarily a professional counselor, but a trusted friend, a spouse, fellow employee, clergy, parent or child. However, don't discount a professional if the need is there. Get whatever helps you need to realign your life's goals, values and dreams. Remember, nothing is worth the ruination of your health.

REPRIORITIZING AND REALISTIC GOAL SETTING

When we first start out in our adult life our priorities might be something like this:
1. Profession or job
2. Money
3. Acquiring property and material goods
4. Family
5. Avocations and recreation
6. Nationality, politics
7. Religion
8. Health

When we get older they may realign themselves more like:
1. Family
2. Health
3. Religion

> ## Always let your physician know what the other is doing!

4. Avocation and recreation
5. Profession or job
6. Money
7. Acquiring property and material goods
8. Nationality, politics

That's quite a change around. Often we are so busy chasing after our goals that we don't even realize they've changed. We should take time out every few years and examine ourselves to adjust our goals to fit our new needs and dreams. If we don't make adjustments, we find distress will rise in every facet of our lives. Have you ever noticed how well adjusted most of those people are who change professions every few years. We tend to look at them as unstable, lost, irresponsible and generally unsuccessful. Take another hard look at them. They probably spend a lot more time smiling than you do. Distress is not a big factor in their lives. They adjust to their needs by changing directions, trying new things, making fresh beginnings. They cope well. They are survivors. They aren't anchored to rigid goals.

Spend a few days listing your <u>real</u> priorities in their proper order. Don't hesitate to move things around in several different orders. Nothing is etched in stone. Let us suggest you place health and recreation high on your list. Both are powerful distress and anger reducers.

RECREATION

We've already mentioned recreation several times, but it deserves a place of its own in this program. Quality recreation time is a must for you. It should be providing the good times for which you live. Quality recreation is one of the best vehicles to strengthen your family relationships. It will help you solve your problems and thus reduce your distress and anger levels. Quality recreation is a powerful method of reducing hypertension.

WHAT IS QUALITY RECREATION?

It is different for each of us. For you, it is the avocation you most enjoy. I emphasize the word "avocation." If you happen to be one of those lucky people who work in a profession or job you truly love to do more than anything else in the world, you still need some form of recreation. You have to be able to get away to something else. It's what prevents job burnout—and you can burn out on any job no matter how terrific it may be to you.

Find avocations you can really throw yourself into. Try to become dedicated to them. If golf is your thing take the challenge and work at becoming the best golfer you can be. If painting or sculpture is it for you, you don't have to become another Grandma Moses or Picasso, but work at becoming the best artist you can be. If you can't get hooked enough, seek out other avocations.

You can't have too many and eventually one will grab you. It has to be able to push your problems right out of your mind. It has to push its way right into "priority one" while you're engaged in its activities. Thus, an avocation that requires skill development and concentration on detail is all the better. In seeking avocations best suited to you, try several activities and continue with those that best turn you on. Perhaps a good place to start is to think about some of the things you wanted to do when you were younger but thought you didn't have the time or finances to pursue. If you can't think of a niche for yourself, the following may help:

EXERCISE....

We've already learned that exercise is the best distress reducer. If you can find an avocation which requires vigorous body activity, that's all the better. This activity should not take the place of your walking program. It must be in addition to your *daily walking*. Team sports, tennis, golf, hiking, body building, swimming and gardening are all activities that fit into this category. Once your walking program has put you into adequate physical condition and your physician gives you the "go ahead," these are good distress reducing avocations.

TRAVEL....

A vacation is a great revitalizer. The main problem is we can't usually take enough of them. As wonderful as it is to get away for two weeks or longer, frequent long weekends are probably better for us. When we come back from very long vacations, the distress caused by all the catching up we have to do may undo all the good our vacation did us. If you only get two weeks vacation, ten working days, you may do better by using them around holiday weekends and getting several four or five day trips a year. If you have a job that requires a lot of travel, consider taking a couple of days at the end of your business trip to save on travel costs and take your spouse along.

BOWLING...

Bowlers all over the world will despise me for not placing bowling under exercise, but as an exercise it doesn't build up much of a sweat. However, as a game of skill and a way to get out with people and take your mind off of distressing problems, it has plenty going for it. Bowling is a competitive activity in which you can improve the rest of your life. There are fine points that you can work at which will require complete concentration. You can join a league, adding excitement and good fellowship—or you can just challenge yourself with constant improvement. One thing you have to watch out for in most bowling alleys is the side stream smoke. More and more bowling alleys are now seeing the benefit of starting smoke-free leagues and making part of their lanes non-smoking. If you can't find one of these more progressive places, suggest to the manager he consider this option.

MUSIC...

"Music tames the savage beast!" There may be no truer statement. Perhaps that is why many conductors, composers and musicians can remain active into their late eighties and nineties. Here, we're not suggesting you be only a spectator. You're never too old to take music lessons. Did you ever wish you'd taken up an instrument as a kid? Perhaps you did take lessons but didn't pursue it as far as you'd liked. No better time than the present to remedy that mistake. We know a fifty-eight year old executive who took up the French Horn two years ago and has become quite proficient at it. He has also become involved with Barber Shop singing and travels to national and international competitions. Music has become a real top priority in his life and he'll tell you he's never enjoyed life more.

CAMPING...

This is a fun and challenging way to travel and meet new

and interesting people. You can back pack in (after your walking program puts you into adequate physical condition) or you can drive to the thousands of campgrounds throughout the world. You can buy or rent a recreational vehicle and have the freedom of a modern day Gypsy. You might try taking a wilderness course to develop some real survival skills. Once you can break the bonds of hotels and motels, the world really becomes yours with limitless frontiers to explore.

CARPENTRY...

If you are talented with your hands and have a creative tendency, consider carpentry or model building. What can be more satisfying as-well-as distress reducing than to see your own creations come to life as you build with wood and tools. This is an avocation in which you will constantly improve and develop new skills. And if woods don't turn you on, perhaps metals will. We know an executive from a large wrecking company who one day started welding together bits and pieces of junk and today is a sculptor of note. His avocation opened whole new vistas to him as he travels to showings of his "works."

PAINTING...

Water color, oils, acrylics, chalk, crayons, pencils or ink and charcoal, all await you to give them a try. You may never sell a picture, but that isn't the main purpose. There are few activities that can be more absorbing than to dabble in paint, color, form.... You don't have to possess great talent to enjoy art. A few lessons and you'll be able to express yourself surprisingly well on paper or canvas. Art skills can be learned to a point where they become at least self-satisfying and totally absorbing—and that's the main idea. But don't be surprised if you discover a real hidden talent, once you give your creativity a chance to nurture.

SCULPTURE...

Who didn't enjoy modeling clay as a child? Why not try the adult version. Sculpture, ceramics, origami, welding, carving, paper mache are just a few of the ways for you to create in three dimensions.

READING...

No matter what other avocation you may choose, there are times when nothing beats a good book. Create time for yourself to get through some of those books you didn't have time for in the past. You might want to join a Great Books group and share your love for literature with new friends. And if good books are your passion, you may want to expand into collecting rare books. Also consider doing volunteer work for your local library association.*

*The Cartographer
*The Remnant
*Shtetl

WRITING...

As writers, we can tell you first hand, there is no more forgiving art form than writing. Anyone can do it! And just about everyone has said at one time or another, "I'd like to write a book about...." Well, there's no time like the present to get started. Writing will completely absorb your mind. You can't do it and worry about anything else that could be causing you distress. If nothing else, write your family history to hand down to your kids and grandkids. But if you have the least desire to write something else—a book, articles, poetry, lyrics,

> Remember, the best distress reducing avocation is one that takes a lot of concentration, demanding that you get your mind off of everything else.

scripts—have at it! The more you write, the more your writing will improve and the more pleasure you'll get from it.*

*So You Want To Write A Book

GARDENING...

A friend of ours who lives in an apartment *(with no yard space)* is one of the most avid gardeners we've ever met. His apartment is a virtual greenhouse. Every window sill, shelf and table has potted plants. He has more plants on his floor than most of us have in our gardens. I often wonder what he'd do if he had a yard. The point is that gardening can be a wonderful avocation and anyone can get into it. You can get started with just a few pots and plants or even seeds. Gardening can be scaled to your own space and needs. There is no end to how far you can take this hobby. You can specialize in orchids, roses, cacti, succulents, wild flowers, herbs, vegetables, trees, fruits, shrubs, or you can go for it all. You can even breed your own varieties. Get a little dirt under your nails and give it a fair try.

FARMING...

If gardening isn't enough of a challenge for you, perhaps you'd like to be a weekend farmer. At first, we thought this a little far fetched, but then we were surprised to find that a lot of city folks have a few acres in the country that they own or rent for horses, cattle turkeys, chickens, rabbits, sheep, goats, pigs, dogs, cats and other critters. Some people grow fruits and vegetables and trees. Some just fish their streams or ponds. If you don't want to raise anything, perhaps just having a weekend home or a private place to camp on a few acres will take your mind off of the distressing factors in your life.

INVESTING...

To me investing has always been a distressing activity, but that's probably because we tend to invest more than we can afford to lose. we envy those who know what they are doing and come up winners. The fact is, if investing isn't what you do for a living and you can afford to take the plunge, it can be an excellent avocation. If you are the type who enjoys researching companies, knows the ins and outs of the markets, can afford the gamble, then investing can be a legitimate hobby for you. This is especially true if your investments include coins, stamps, art, antiques....

ENTREPRENEURSHIP...

If you qualify for the investing hobby category, then this is just a step beyond. Just don't get into something that adds to your distress!*

*Secrets to Creating Passive Income

VOLUNTEER WORK...

Perhaps there is no more satisfying a avocation than volunteer work. Helping others who are less fortunate has its own rewards. It's a way of paying back for our own good fortune and blessings. It can be done in any degree and there is no end to organizations who need your help. Churches, synagogues, hospitals, service organizations, schools, the Red Cross, the Salvation Army, the Peace Corps, Vista, local and international groups, the Boy and Girl Scouts are but a few who need your help and expertise. Try giving a few hours of yourself a week and see what it does to your distress and anger levels. You are a valuable commodity and resource and you owe it to yourself and your community—your world—to share yourself with others.*

*The Joy of Volunteering

HIKING....

If you are near the woods, mountains, lakes, rivers, the countryside or anywhere else that lends itself to hiking, then by all means hike. It's an avocation in which you can participate with your spouse, the whole family, grandchildren and friends. On a hiking day, you needn't take your daily walk. Just hike further, longer, a little slower and enjoy it more. Look and listen. Notice the animals and birds, plants and trees. Even insects can be fascinating. Observe nature and try to learn about it. Here's an opportunity to slow down and see things that you've been too busy and in too much of a rush to enjoy in years past.*

*The Second Half Begins at 50

TEACHING....

In all the years you've lived and experienced, you've learned a lot more than you realize. You have skills and knowledge that others can and want to learn from. Teaching is one of the most satisfying and fun experiences imaginable. Check around your local schools and universities. Many have adult continuing education programs that offer any number of courses from ballroom dancing to word processing, bookkeeping, languages, entrepreneurship to writing. We bet you've had an interesting enought life that you have something quite worthwhile to pass on to others. Look upon it is as an obligation to share your expertise with others. And if you really can't find something that you can teach to others, then consider taking some courses and broadening your horizons.

GOLF....

Golf, like bowling, deserves special mention. It has little aerobic exercise value, but it is a skill activity that constantly challenges one and is an excellent hobby. It takes you out of doors, expands your friendships, is something you can do with friends and acquaintances, is mind absorbing and does help you to stay physically limber. If you can walk the course, all the better. And you're never too old to take it up or play. Our mother, in her nineties and after her open heart surgery still played weekly.

FISHING....

Fishing is an international pastime. You can practice this art anywhere in the world. From trolling to fly casting to deep sea fishing and spear fishing, it's always a challenge. You can get a workout fishing or you can snooze on the bank of a stream or lake waiting for a strike, but whichever you do, it is a good distress reducing activity. Fishing is a great family avocation or you can sneak off by yourself if solitude is what you need most.

FLYING....

This is a rich man's or woman's hobby, but if you can afford it, flying is an adventure in itself. There is powered aircraft or you can go in for gliding if you live where there are good air currents and thermal. If you're real adventurous you might even go in for ballooning or hang gliding. This is certainly not for everyone, but if it's something you've always wanted to do—why not now?

BOATING....

Boating is among the world's most practiced pastimes. You can spend millions on a yacht or just a few hundred bucks on a canoe. We'll never forget the sign we saw on a yacht docked in the Bahamas, "The greatest two days in a boat owner's life are the day he buys his boat—and the day he sells it!" What the sign didn't tell me was that most boat owners sell their boats only to turn around and buy a bigger boat!

PHOTOGRAPHY....

Photography is an activity that works in combination with almost any other hobby you might choose. With today's amazing and amazingly inexpensive automatic cameras, almost anyone can be an expert photographer. Digital cameras and technology has made photography much more versatile for amateurs since now it is easier to do your own finishing and altering or tweaking and printing your photos with your computer and printer. And with the easy-to-use video cameras you can even be your own movie producer.

LEARNING....

There are a vast array of adult education courses offered by public schools, colleges, churches, synagogues, organizations, museums, galleries and private institutions, you can study almost anything you want. Learning in itself is a wonderful hobby, but more importantly, it can introduce you to many other exciting activities and interests to pursue in the future. The old adage, "You can't teach an old dog new tricks," isn't true. the problem is that too many of us "old dogs" just don't try. Put forth the effort and you can learn anything you want and the more you learn the easier it becomes.*

* **Sharpening the Aging Mind**

STAMP COLLECTING....

This is a hobby you can apply yourself to in all degrees. Perhaps you want to limit yourself to stamps of one type, like sports stamps from all countries, or stamps from all the places you've visited—or maybe you want to go in for investing in rare stamps. This avocation can be limited to your kitchen table or it can take you all over the world to stamp shows and conventions.

DANCING....

Ballroom dancing is making a real comeback with competitions and clubs popping up everywhere. Or maybe you just want to be able to "cut a mean rug" once in a while at parties or on nights out. Perhaps you'd like to get into a tap dancing class. Dancing is a very healthy avocation, giving you a good workout while taking your mind off of disturbing factors in your life. Dancing lessons are readily available most everywhere.

BIKING....

If you have good bike paths available to you give it a try. It doesn't take the place of your daily walking, but it makes an excellent additional activity. You should be able to rent a bike to give it a fair trial before investing in your own. Bicycles aren't cheap anymore and the technology has changed considerably since the last time you rolled up your pant leg and took a turn.

COLLECTING....

Collecting anything, stamps, coins, art, antiques, old cars, rare books, whatever strikes your fancy, can be a wonderful avocation. Collecting can take you to all corners of the world, or it can bring the world to you. You'll meet other people with similar interests to yours and you might find yourself owning some real treasures. Most important the study, travel and challenge of collecting will go a long way to reducing the distress of your daily life.

This listing is just a scratch in the surface of all the leisure time activities you can get involved in. The most important thing is that you get involved. Don't limit yourself to just one avocation. The more you engage in, the broader your interests will be and the better, more relaxed you'll be for it. Above all, learn to enjoy life. Reprioritize! The things that you've let distress you all of your life probably were never as important as you made them. We create most of our distress—and we can rid ourselves of distress with just a little effort—and fun!

Resources mentioned in this chapter include:

SO YOU WANT TO WRITE A BOOK - THORNTON PUBLISHING - 2008   ISBN: 0-9801941-3-X

Othniel Seiden, MD & Jane L. Bilett, Ph.D.

THE JOY OF VOLUNTEERING - THORNTON PUBLISHING - 2008 - BOOMER BOOK SERIES COMING IN 2008

THE CARTOGRAPHER..1492 - THORNTON PUBLISHING 2007 BOOMER BOOK SERIES ISBN: 0-9801941-2-1

THE REMNANT - THORNTON PUBLISHING - 2008 BOOMER BOOK SERIES ISBN: 0-9801941-4-8

SHETTL - THORNTON PUBLISHING - 2011 BOOMER BOOK SERIES ISBN: 0-9801941-4-8

SECRETS TO CREATING PASSIVE INCOME - THORNTON PUBLISHING 2008 BOOKS TO BELIEVE IN ISBN: 0-9801941-9-9

CHAPTER 11

YOUR MOTIVES REVISITED...

If this program fails for you it is not because you can't stick to it or that it won't work for you; rather, *it's because you're not motivated enough!* Motivation makes the difference. If you aren't dedicated enough to make the simple lifestyle changes required, then you'll fail for sure. However, if your health means enough to you to make and stick by the few simple changes, then your success is assured.

You must have some motivation to get back into shape else you wouldn't have bought this book. Of course, "get back into shape," presupposes that you once were in shape. That's not necessarily true. Most Americans are far out of shape and have been that way since childhood.

We really aren't the least interested in your past. It's from this day forward that interests us. Follow the program in this book, and a year from now you can be in the best condition you've been in, in years—regardless of age. And the only thing which might be standing in the way is lack of motivation, so let's build on the bit of motivation that got you to buy this book and read this far between its covers.

One of the strongest motivations for you to get into and stay in shape is that if you don't, it's a downhill slide for you from this point to the grave. Your choice is either you make an effort to improve yourself, or next year at this time—and every succeeding year—you're going to be fatter, flabbier, weaker, with less endurance, resistance and appeal to others.

We can't keep you from aging, but the process can be slowed. Your physical aging need not speed ahead of your chronological age or even keep up with it. No one can guarantee you'll live any longer because you're in good shape and physical condition, but authorities on aging and longevity all bet you will. We'll guarantee you'll enjoy the rest of your life a lot more if you maintain your physical and mental health— and that is what this book is really all about.

Getting into your best possible physical condition will require four main activities; correcting your nutritional status, establishing your walking program, reducing your stress/distress ratio and getting rid of a few bad habits you may have picked up along the way which we will deal with later. To do these things, you'll have to establish some goals. Setting goals is not that difficult and this book will help you to set realistic targets for yourself. Continuing to work toward those goals is, however, another matter. Motivation is what will spell your success or failure. Keeping you on the straight and narrow in the corrected direction is our main purpose. The good news is that good habits are not that hard to form and after a few weeks of your "new lifestyle" it will become second nature to you and better than what you are living now. In other words, if you can motivate yourself to stick to your new lifestyle long enough for it to become "habit," the rest will be easy.

To help you through these first few weeks think of all the reasons you might want to get into better physical condition. Make a list that you can review each day. Add to the list as new reasons suggest themselves. If you have trouble thinking of some reasons let me suggest a few.

YOU'D LIKE TO LOOK BETTER...

We can't think of anyone who doesn't want to look more attractive. Anyone who says this reason isn't close to the top of his/her list of motives is probably kidding him/herself. It is a rare person who cares nothing about his/her appearance. This is one of the strongest motivating forces to get one into good physical condition.

Your appearance establishes the first impression when others meet you. Others draw immediate opinions about you the instant they see you, before you say a word to show them what a stunning mind and personality you really have. If you make a poor appearance, your job of winning them over is that much more difficult, be it social, business or family situations. Consider how much easier it would be to attract others to yourself, your ideas, your projects, your bed if you were at or near your ideal body weight.

YOU'D LIKE TO FEEL BETTER...

Remember how much more energy you had five or ten years ago? Or maybe it was just last year? Last month? If you don't turn things around, think how rotten you'll feel next year or in five years. Either you're going to feel better than ever next year—or you're going to be another year older and feel a couple years older or worse. It's not going to get better unless you do something about it now and keep on working at it. If you improve your physical condition during this year, you'll begin to feel better and continue to feel better and better as time goes on. If, on the other hand, you continue in the direction you've been headed, you can expect to become a bigger and pudgier than ever.

Along with improved nutritional status, activity, endurance, muscle tone, reduction of fat deposits will come feelings of well being and energy you never thought you'd experience again.

YOU'D LIKE TO BECOME A BETTER ATHLETE...

Your aspirations don't have to be toward world class competition; there are a lot of reasons to want to become more proficient at athletic activities you enjoy. If you improve your game, whatever it is, golf, bowling, racquet ball, tennis, touch football, whatever, you'll have more fun at it. Athletics doesn't mean you have to join a team, league or expensive athletic club. Maybe you just want to be able to keep up with your kids—or parents!

YOU'D LIKE TO TONE UP...

Being a proficient athlete may be low on your priority list. How about just firming up those loose muscles and trimming off a lot of that storage fat along the way. If nothing else it will give you a better body to hang your clothes on. It won't happen unless you get off your butt and on your feet a little more. Remember, you're not being asked to run a daily military obstacle course, just to take a brisk walk five or more days a week.

If you alter your nutritional habits a little and walk an hour a day for just five days a week you'll remove about a pound of storage fat from your body each week. Think that isn't a lot? Go out into the kitchen and see how big a one pound can of cooking fat or butter is. A pound of cooking lard and your lard are about the same in volume and quality. Now imagine how much better you'll feel when about twenty-five of those come off your body mass.

YOU NEED TO LOSE SOME WEIGHT FOR THE BUSINESS...

There is no doubt that you'll meet the public better, earn the respect of colleagues easier and impress your superiors more, if you look better and have more energy, vigor and endurance. You'll do a better job no matter what it is. If you don't do work that requires strength and action, remember

> It's never too late to get into good shape even if you've never been there before!

that a mind in a healthy body functions better, clearer, faster, more efficiently and longer.

Still need more convincing? Well, ask yourself this question, "If there are two of us trying out for the same position or promotion and we're equally capable in all respects, but the other guy looks a lot sharper—who's going to get the job?"

Being able to earn more money can be a strong motivator!

YOU'RE TIRED OF BREAKING DOWN...

It's a fact that as your body deteriorates, it loses its resistance to bacteria, viruses, sprains, strains, stresses and other maladies. You might just as well face it, your body is going to continue to deteriorate until you make a concerted effort to turn things around. There's no such thing as status quo in biology. You have to choose between working at getting better and healthier or watching yourself go to pot. If you choose the spectator role you'll see yourself get fatter, weaker, more prone to illness, developing aches and pains and generally turning more unattractive and uninteresting as a person.

It's your choice!

YOU WANT TO SCORE BETTER WITH THE OPPOSITE SEX...

Sex is of some importance to everyone, damned important to most of us. Some won't admit it as eagerly as others. If you're married, you want your spouse to feel proud of you. A stronger way to put it is, *you don't want you spouse to be ashamed to be seen with you!* If you're married you still want others of the opposite sex to take positive note of you. If you're married and you don't care how your spouse thinks about you, then we'd bet you are even more concerned over how others of the opposite sex see you! Put simply, if you're one of the less than 50% of our population that is faithful to his/her mate, then you want that mate to "get a buzz" when he or she is with you. If you're one of the more than 50% of our population, who is not faithful to your mate, then you'll probably want someone else to "get a buzz" when he or she is with you.

Of course if you're not married you probably want to make everyone "buzz!" We're really not interested in your morality; we just want to tell you, if you want to be attractive to others your job will be easier if you get into shape! If you're among the 10 or 20 percent of our population who doesn't care whether it is the opposite sex, the same still goes. Sexual fantasies are strong motivations. *People who are healthy, as-well-as in good shape, are just more attractive to everyone.*

YOU WANT TO BE STRONGER...

Remember the old Charles Atlas ads? They sold a lot of self-improvement courses. Why? It's because we all want to feel more confident. It wasn't just the bulging muscles, but what those muscles represented. We want to be strong though very few of us have a goal of being a body builder. For those who want that, great! Go for it! For most of us, however, added strength really adds to our confidence. As your body improves so will your self-image which builds your confidence.

As your body builds muscle tone, it becomes harder for others to take advantage of you, push you around or kick sand in your face. Not because they will be scared you'll punch them in the nose, but because you'll exude new confidence and people don't try to intimidate those who exude confidence.

YOU WANT TO GAIN WEIGHT...

People like you drive people like us nuts. You eat and we gain weight! People who look like slobs envy you who look like bean poles, but we're sure you are every bit as distressed about your shape as we are. Your underweight problem is every bit as difficult to deal with as our overweight.

Most people who want to gain weight try to put it on by eating. Two things are wrong with that plan. First, your metabolism is probably so elevated that you'll never build any storage fat. Second, fat is not the kind of weight you want to add. Remember, fat doesn't weigh nearly as much as muscle or lean meat. You get muscle by exercising, not just by eating. You should look into a body building program in addition to your walking program.

YOU WANT YOUR FRIENDS AND FAMILY TO RESPECT YOU...

Peer regard is perhaps the strongest motivator there is. What our friends and close acquaintances think of us is extremely important. We play different roles to our friends because we want their respect in specific ways. If they can respect our physical prowess and appearance, it is a plus to the relationship. Self-esteem depends on the esteem of others. You can't think highly of yourself if you don't think others think well of you. Your wife and kids and grandchildren will think better of you if you aren't a weak, sickly, inactive milk-toast!

YOU WANT PRAISE INSTEAD OF CRITICISM...

If you've been "overweight" and out of shape for some time, We're sure you've heard your share of unkind comments—some from well-meaning persons, others form those less kind finding a place to dig at you where it hurts. Just as criticism is punishing to us, so is praise a reward. Reward is a much stronger motivating tool than punishment of criticism. If you're finally sick to death of the criticism, perhaps your quest for praise will drive you to the decision to improve your physical condition. Praise will drive most people to higher aspiration.

YOU WANT TO LOOK YOUNGER...

Humankind has been dreaming of the fountain of youth since ancient times. Of course, eternal youth is beyond even the scope of this book, but renewed vigor, improved appearance, revitalized strength and health are not. And those are the characteristics that do spell a more youthful appearance and self-esteem. Going to seed does indeed overemphasize aging. Get back into shape and people will comment that you are looking younger. You'll feel younger, function younger— and if it makes you live longer that's almost the same as being younger. In other words, we are trying to do both—*put more years into your life and a lot more life into your years!*

YOU WANT TO BELONG TO THE "IN" GROUP—THE HEALTHY PEOPLE...

To be part of a group, a movement, or to be included and affiliated are all strong motivating forces. The human animal is a social creature. Most of us gravitate to groups of people with like interests. Birds of a feather do indeed flock together. Right now, you may belong to a sedentary group of dodo birds. Well, if you'll recall, the dodo bird was a large, flightless bird and has been extinct since the 17th century. And in today's society the sedentary pudgies are also becoming an extinct group. They are literally dying off at a faster rate than the more "in" group, the slimmer, trimmer, more active group. If you're normal you will want to "fly with the eagles" rather than wander toward extinction with the dodo birds. The "in" group is having all the fun while the pudgies don't have a whole lot going for them.

YOUR SPOUSE IS ON YOUR CASE...

Most people are very concerned about their spouse's health, appearance and welfare. That's why they want them to do something positive about their physical shape and health. Who can blame them? The prospect of widow or widower hood is not usually a bright one. If you won't shape up for yourself—maybe you'll do it for him or her.

These are but a few of the reasons people give for finally deciding to get back into shape. Whatever your reasons may be, don't let them get away from you. Write them down. Keep them where you can see them easily, where you can look at them often to remind yourself. Any reason should be reason enough. Review the reasons above and add your own reasons in the space below:

_____

_____

_____

_____

_____

_____

_____

Remember, motivation is all that stands between you and your success in this program!

CHAPTER 12

INCREASE YOUR
CHANCES...

In the beginning of this book, we stated that the human body was designed to survive in good working order for at least 120 years. Obviously few of us are reaching that potential. We've malnourished ourselves, poisoned ourselves, misused ourselves, let ourselves run down, distressed ourselves . . . *but* in spite of all that, 75,000 of us will be living to over 100 years in just a half decade from now, and that number increases at a dizzying rate. This chapter will give you a few hints at things you can do in addition to the fore-mentioned lifestyle changes, just to tip the odds in your favor to be among those passing their one century birthday . . . and enjoying the party!

Remember the statistic; in spite of the fact that, in the past decades American's life spans have lengthened dramatically, *American's longevity is only forty-second in the world,* and many of those countries ahead of us are Third World! There is plenty of room for our improvement!

The fore mentioned lifestyle changes are for the most part prevention techniques. They keep us from doing damage to your body which can shorten its potential longevity. The following are for the most part survival techniques. They put the odds towered helping you survive dread illnesses should they befall you. Some are also preventative as well as reducing your chances of succumbing, should your new preventive lifestyle not have started quite in time. Discuss them with your medical advisors should any of these measures be contra-indicated in your situation.

ASA -- Acetylsalicylic Acid -- Plain ol', aspirin!

Aspirin is among our oldest medications. It is without a doubt the most versatile and amazing medical discovery in history. Our parents, our grandparents, most likely our great-grandparents took it for fever and pain, colds, flu, chills, strains and sprains and for almost everything else if nothing specific was available. And in most cases it helped. We are just finding out in our time how remarkable this medication really is.

If we could only give one piece of medical advice to people, the following sentence would probably be the one we'd choose, because we feel it will save and prolong more lives than any other advice or medical procedure in our armamentarium of medical skills. That's a profound opinion, but we believe it.

Ask your medical advisor about it. I believe, Why? It's because one aspirin a day can increase your chances of surviving a heart attack by 47%. In addition, it dramatically reduces the chances of having that heart attack. It dramatically reduces the chances of having a stroke and it reduces the chances of a stroke from leaving permanent damage and reduces the seriousness of that permanent damage should it persist. Aspirin is linked to the prevention of several cancers and may slow or help prevent the onset of Alzheimer disease. It retards the onset of inflammatory diseases and the permanent damage they can do such as arthritis and joint diseases.

If aspirin tends to irritate your stomach, ask your medical

advisor about enteric coated or buffered aspirin. *Remember, if you are allergic to aspirin, if you have a bleeding problem or if you take blood thinning or other incompatible medication, you are among the few who should not take one aspirin daily! Check with your personal medical advisor before starting any medication that you intend taking on a permanent basis.*

Anti-Oxidants

Anti-Oxidants are getting lots of press these days. These are vitamins which reduce the cellular damage or certain carcinogens that circulate in our bodies. Among these are Alpha-carotene, Vitamins C, E, the hormone Melatonin and several other less important. Melatonin is naturally occurring in the body, produced by the pineal gland. As we age, the secretion of Melatonin is reduced, so some physicians are advising supplementation in pill form. We have no way of measuring at what point if ever Melatonin levels drop to a level which requires supplementation. As far as anyone knows, however, Melatonin supplementation has no detrimental effect. It has not been studied for a very long period of time, but people who have taken it for many years have shown no ill effects. It is reported to have anti-aging properties in animals but human studies have not yet declared it the fountain of youth. It does work in reducing jet lag and for some sleep problems seems to work wonders. Very low doses of Melatonin are adequate, probably 1 to 3 mg daily or less. It should be taken only under the direction of *your personal physician* and the longer it is taken the lower the dose is needed.

Alpha-Carotene, Vitamins C and E and most other anti-oxidants are readily found in fruits and vegetables. Proper nutrition should provide you with all you need, but most of us fail in proper nutrition, so as we age and start to eat a little less properly, supplementation won't hurt. Alpha-Carotene is in the vitamin A group and one of the few vitamins which can be overdosed. You should not take over 25,000 units of Alpha-Carotene per day. Vitamin E 400 mg and C at 1000 mg should be sufficient supplementation for most of us who eat healthy.

Do we take the above mentioned supplements?

All but Melatonin!

Geriatric dentistry

Now that we are getting older there's a new kid in town, the geriatric dentist. Yes, it's a new specialty. Does it mean we have to leave our old dentist? Not necessarily. He or she will probably take some special courses or study up on the new problems age brings to dentistry. The important thing is that you know there are some new problems on the horizon. Ask your dentist about them and what you can do to prevent them.

Among other things we have a reduction in salivation as we age. Especially at night our mucous membranes tend to dry leaving that horrible taste in our mouths. Saliva also tends to keep our teeth and gums healthy, rinsing them and reducing bacteria.

Some of us will lose some of our dexterity in brushing. That will also tend to reduce our oral hygiene and give dental and gum disease a foothold. The electric tooth brush is a real boon to the elderly who have a tendency to get lazy or just lose the agility required for good brushing.

Mandibular recession is another problem we face as we age. The bones holding the teeth in place tend to reabsorb and lose some of their mineral calcium. Calcium supplement may be effective in slowing this problem. Recession of the gums is another problem, especially with drying of the mucus membranes and less effective brushing. As the gums recede, we are subject to root damage and decay. There are a couple of preventive measures here. Floss, floss, floss! Good flossing of the teeth will reduce the impacted foods between the teeth and gums that nurture bacterial growth and plaque. Fluoride becomes important again as we age, to prevent damage to teeth and roots. Fluoride rinses are quite effective as are fluoride tooth pastes.

As our populations age, dental implants will become more common. This procedure is replacing dentures and bridge work rapidly. Hopefully the procedure will become less costly and time consuming as it is perfected. In the mean time, take good care of your oral hygiene so that implants can be avoided. **Discuss your dental future with your dentist!** If you have any dental problems get them taken care of **now!**— before they lead to more difficult problems and have a chance to effect your general health!

"Anyone over the age of 30 years, who is not allergic to aspirin or on a blood thinning medication, should take one aspirin daily under his or her personal medical advisor's direction.

Immunizations....

The elderly often have more difficulty overcoming illnesses. Furthermore, serious and prolonged illnesses can start a downward spiral in our total well being. Any time we can take steps to prevent such illnesses we should take advantage of them. Immunizations are one way of protecting our well being and health.

Flu Vaccine

Every fall and winter flu kills thousands of elderly people in the United States who could have been protected by a simple injection. Contrary to what people say, almost always those who don't take the shot, flu vaccine is very unlikely to make you sick.

Get a flu vaccine every fall!

Hepatitis A and B

These vaccines have become recently available. They are relatively expensive, but the diseases they protect you from are potentially lethal and hospitalization and lost time is far more expensive. Hopefully travel will be an important part of your retirement years and if foreign travel makes up any part of that, these immunizations are all the more important. Enjoy the Sushi!

Meningococcal meningitis

This vaccine is available and protects against infection which can cause permanent central nervous system and brain damage and death.

Streptococcal pneumonia

This is a vaccine which gives lifelong protection to this potentially fatal lung disease which too frequently brings about the early demise of the elderly.

Tetanus/Diphtheria

Also known as DipTet, it should be injected every ten years, and anytime a deep contaminated puncture wound is acquired such as a bite or dirty nail piercing.

Typhoid

This is an important vaccine, especially if you'll be traveling. This is now available orally and thought to be more effective than the shot..

Endemic diseases

These are diseases which are prevalent in certain areas of the world where you may be traveling. You should contact the **Center for Disease Control (CDC) at 404-332-4559** before any trip to inquire about regional endemic health problems and the immunizations and precautions you can take to protect yourself. These may include **Polio, Yellow Fever, Malaria, Cholera** and other exotic diseases. With proper protection and information, you should never have to fear travel and new experiences.

JUST FOR THE LADIES....

There is no truth to the myth that Pap smears and pelvic examinations are no longer necessary after menopause. Ovarian, uterine and cervical cancers kill too many women and these are detectable and successfully treatable in most cases through timely examinations. Gynecologic examinations must be a yearly habit for every woman regardless of age. Forgetting is no excuse. Being too busy is no excuse. Let a birthday or anniversary remind you every year and do it a day before or after. Make a mammogram part of that same examination. Breast cancer can strike at any age and early discovery gives you a high chance for cure. If you do not do self breast exams once a month, ask your medical advisor to show you how and **do it on the first day of each month!** *When I was in private practice I taught husbands or partners to check their partner's breasts once a month ... it got done more often and regularly that way.* Your doctor can teach your partner to do the exam.

Calcium supplementation is of particular important to women, especially after menopause, to prevent osteoporosis and compression fractures though these problems do occur in men far less frequently. Supplementation should begin in the 30s or 40s, but if you are past that age and haven't started, calcium supplementation should start today! If you drink lots of milk (skim) and or eat lots of cottage cheese (low fat) you may not need supplementation, but most women don't get sufficient calcium in their diets. Talk to your pharmacist or medical adviser to determine the best calcium supplement for you. Other medications available to fight and even reverse the bone loss of osteoporosis are estrogen therapy, Calcitonin, Sodium Fluoride and Alendronate (Fosomax). Discuss these therapies with your medical advisor.

Heart disease has been too long ignored in women. *Heart disease is the number one killer of women.* When we didn't live as long as we now do women didn't develop heart disease as early as men and it was thought they weren't as susceptible. That has changed, but the myth remains. In the post menopausal years women develop heart disease at a more rapid rate then men and in their late sixties and seventies are very susceptible to heart attack and failure especially now that they are smoking in such great numbers. Let me repeat, *Heart Disease is the number one killer* of women. Estrogen therapy is one method of prolonging their pre-menopausal protection. Also quit smoking right now if you indulge, exercise and reduce your ingestion of saturated fats. Insist on the same cardiac attention from your medical advisor as he would give to a male your age. Also, it must be remembered that women do not always have the same "classic" heart attack symptoms as a man. Women may have their pain in the back between the scapulas; they may not have the perspiration or the radiation of pain to the neck and left arm.

If these classic signs do appear **get to an emergency**

room via a 911 call as quickly as possible.
*Heart of a Woman

JUST FOR THE MEN....

Two problems men must watch for, one unique, the other more prevalent to them, are **Prostate problems and cancer and Rectal cancer.** Prostrate problems include infections and **benign prostatic hypertrophy (BPH).** Benign Prostatic Hypertrophy is a non-cancerous enlargement of the prostate gland which almost all men have as they age. In an appreciable number of men, this growth of the gland causes some degree of obstruction to the normal flow of urine from the bladder to excretion. There are some medications now available to relieve this obstruction without having to resort to surgery. They are worth trying. If, however they do not work, surgical intervention may be required to prevent complete obstruction. These can include removal of the gland, boring out a portion of the gland along the urethra or tube which allows the flow of urine, using microwave to shrink the gland or placing a stint in the urethra or spreading it (not unlike angioplasty) to keep it open.

Prostate cancer is a growing problem as men live longer. Fortunately it is a very slow growing cancer in most cases and early detection offers a high percentage of cures. The key word is **"early!"** There are two main methods of screening for prostate cancer. One is the blood test **PSA**, the other is yearly rectal examination of the prostate. Both of these tests should be carried out on every male over the age of 45. If either is indicative of suspicion of prostate cancer, they should be followed up with an ultra sound examination and possibly a needle biopsy of the prostate. If these are negative, great! Live on! If these are positive! You've caught it early! **Treat and live on!**

*Coping with BPH
*Coping with Prostate Cancer

Rectal and colon cancer are certainly not unique to men but more prevalent than in women. Both should be checked yearly for signs of the disease, especially men. Again, the best chance for a high incidence of cure is **"early detection!"** Early detection depends on a simple test for blood in your stools. It should be a yearly check.

For a long healthy life, it is essential that you keep the good health you have now, take care of any problems that presently exist, and do all you can to discover any new problems in time to correct them. This requires a team effort between you and your dentist, pharmacist and medical advisors.

They can't help you if you don't seek their help or follow their advice.

CHAPTER 13

YOUR LIFESTYLE... GETTING WHAT YOU REALLY WANT OUT OF LIFE...

This program is all about your lifestyle and those positive changes you can make to give you a happier, fuller, healthier and longer active presence on this planet. Emphasis is on your lifestyle, and no one else's. To be the healthiest and happiest person you can be, all goals must be set by you. No one else can determine how you should live your life. You have to make it fit the needs of your family, loved ones and close friends. You can't just run roughshod over them ignoring their needs for your own gratification. But within the bounds of what your family and society demand of you, there is a great leeway which you can function happily and healthily.

If you are the breadwinner for your family, that is an obligation you must fulfill, but there are a lot of ways in which you can win bread. The amount of bread necessary is also quite variable. You and your family and those who depend on you must determine just what your real needs, values and goals should be. You might feel it is up to you to earn as much money for your family as is humanly possible for you. It may surprise you to discover that your family would be happier if you'd bring home a little, maybe a lot less, money if it would mean they could spend more time with you.

If you're unhappy with your work but feel you couldn't earn quite as much if you changed jobs, you might find out that your family would rather you earn a little less and be happy with what you are doing. After all, if you're happier at work you'll be happier at home, less distressed, less angry—

ALWAYS REMEMBER...
You are the head
of your own health care team!.

---

and therefore healthier.

And don't let a weight chart or Madison Avenue tell you what you should weigh. That is also a very individual matter. You can be healthy and heavier than those charts demand. If you feel better tipping the scale several pounds heavier with a physique somewhat more round than what the Madison Avenue people show in their ads, that's alright too—as long as you bring your fat to lean body mass into a safe range. Remember, you can do that by bringing up your muscle mass as well as by bringing down your fat tissue. The point is *you and only you* can determine where *your ideal body weight* will eventually be. And you are the one responsible for your health. The best eating habits for you should be determined by you within the confines of what are good nutritional rules. Follow good nutritional habits, emphasizing low fat and high fiber consumption and you should be able to eat happily and healthy for the rest of your life and never d--t again.

Exercise vigorously with an aerobic program fitted to you and you should be healthy regardless of you weight. Keep yourself in line with all the other measures of good health and forget stepping on the scale every morning. That will just cause you needless distress.

If you have any habits that involve destructive chemical abuse get help today!

Then design a lifestyle for yourself that will bring you all the happiness and fulfillment you need.

CHAPTER 14

YOUR SEX LIFE CAN BE BETTER THAN EVER BEFORE AT ANY AGE...

The *Journal of the American Medical Association* in 1999 reported that 4 out of 10 women and 3 out of 10 men claimed some form of sexual dysfunction. The Kinsey Institute stated that 26% of all women in their studies complained of sexual problems and dissatisfaction. The vast majority of women in their studies never reached orgasm through intercourse alone. Saddest of all, 40 million Americans are in sexless marriages. Today's figures state 15% to 20% of marriages are without sexual relationships and many couples have sex less than once per month. Viagra, Levitra and Cialis have not been the panacea expected by many couples who discovered they had a relationship problem rather than a physical erection problem. To us, these are disturbing statistics certainly deserving of a chapter on the subject of "Sex in the Golden Years." (ISBN: 0-9801941-0-5)

Focusing on techniques, priorities, communication and attention to partner's needs can do more for a relationship than pills in many of these cases. Now we realize that most of the readers of this book are not in sexless relationships, in fact, the great majority of you are in situations of better than average sexual gratification but a little tweaking to recapture some of the old spice or add some new tricks to add to an already happy sex life can't hurt.

The purpose of this chapter is to strengthen your relationships and deepen the love and feelings your have for your partner. It should provide you the necessary skills to give your partner the best sexual experiences humanly possible. By doing this, you should achieve the best sex you have ever had. You will learn how to achieve the most frequent and most intense orgasm you've ever experienced. It should rekindle your romance and ignite your love life to an intensity never before achieved. And if you think age is a problem … your future may hold the best sex and loving relationship ever.

What the chapter is not intended to do

This chapter is not intended to *cure* deep seated psychological inhibitions or medical or physical problems that stand in the way of normal sexual function. That must be done by your own medical advisor or someone he or she refers. Our philosophy is that no one or no couple should have to suffer sexual dysfunctions and virtually all such problems can be helped. Since there are serious potential interactions between medications you might be on, or there may be medical problems we can't possibly know about, this type treatment should only be provided by your own medical advisor who knows your entire medical history.

> Your health and your longevity
> are greatly determined by you!

What are your responsibilities?

Pleasing your partner is numero uno! A simple change in attitude for those who have not discovered it yet, is that the best way to achieve the closest relationship, deepest love and most exciting sex is that *your main focus is to give your partner the greatest and most satisfying pleasure possible.*

Pleasure for you should take care of itself if numero uno is ecstatic! If you bring yourself to focus completely on giving your partner intense pleasure, you will quickly discover *it really is better to give than to receive!* A narcissistic individual, one who thinks him or herself the center of the universe; thinking only of the pleasure coming to him or her, is missing out on the truest pleasure of all. We can think of no greater turn-on than having your partner contort, shudder and moan or scream with pleasure and this will lead you to your own greatest pleasure-filled orgasms (and the plural of orgasms is not a typographical error!) Both men and women can learn to have multiple orgasms in their love making, each becoming more intense and delightful than the last! More on male multiple orgasm later, for both of you to look forward to!

LOVE, LUST AND PLEASURE...

The brain is actually the <u>largest</u> and most important <u>sex organ!</u>

The genitals don't hold a candle to the brain when it comes to love and sexuality. You may feel your horniness in the genital area, but it is the brain that turns it all on. Who is attractive to you? How you react to the feelings you get from your attraction? How your attraction reacts to you? What you both do about it -all this is mutual brain work.

The brain is what makes you kind, playful, romantic,

enthusiastic, considerate, committed, and loving to your partner. If dysfunctional, it leads you into impulsive behavior, distraction, unfaithfulness, hatefulness, anger, ruining your chances for real intimacy and a loving relationship. Fortunately, the brain in most cases, is a trainable sex organ, and most sexual dysfunctions are thus correctable with changes in attitudes, training and practice.

Know your own and your partner's special desires and needs

Know your own likes and dislikes. This may require trial and error experimenting alone or together (probably both ways). As important as knowing what stimulation is a turn-on and pleasure giver, is to know what is a turn-off; causing discomfort and anxiety. They should be avoided. With time these dislikes may become less threatening and may even become pleasurable as trust, confidence and emotions deepen. Relationships are dynamic, constantly changing and patience is a strong alley.

Know your partner's likes and dislikes. The more you know about each other's turn-on, joys, delights and needs, the closer and better your relationship will be in all areas. Remember, your major responsibility is to give your partner the greatest pleasure possible. That means to concentrate on the positive and avoid the negative. This is a good philosophy in all aspects of your life together, not just in sex.

Communicating what's good and what's great and what's a no-no!

Feel free to speak your mind and feelings. One of the greatest causes for discord among couples is an inability to communicate. Great communication takes time to develop. It requires building confidence so that what is said will be taken in the proper way, will not have unpleasant repercussions, and will be taken seriously. As a relationship grows stronger, communications tend to improve and as communications improve, relationships grow stronger.

Read your partner's body language for what's too difficult to express verbally. As with verbal communications, recognizing the signals your partner expresses through body language will become more familiar to you. If she moans or screams with delight, you really don't have to ask if she liked it. If he has a stupid grin on his face, you'll know it feels good to him without asking. With time more subtle signs will become more recognizable … pay attention to them.

Ask questions! If he or she doesn't volunteer some information and you can't read the body language, ask. By the same token, if he or she can't read your body language or if there is something you want to change or try, ask. In a successful relationship very few, if any, subjects should be undiscuss-able. Don't expect your partner to be a mind reader!

DELIVERING THE GOODS...

Take care of the things that stand in the way of great relationships and sex.

Hygiene should come before your partner comes. Oral hygiene is a prelude to good old necking. Cleaning teeth should become a habit anytime you even suspect that there might be an intimate encounter. Dental care is essential for sweet kisses and general good health. It's not just that probably no one can be too enthusiastic about kissing an unhealthy mouth full of decay, but poor dental health can lead to an enormous number of general systemic illnesses and diseases which can be life shortening.

If you smoke... QUIT! Unless your partner also smokes, it can't be pleasant getting too close to you, much less kissing you. If your partner also smokes, then you both should quit. Tobacco diminishes sexual drive and performance dramatically. It has a damaging affect on erection, sensation and orgasm. That is not just a problem for the male, but reduces clitoral erection and sensitivity and orgasm for females. We won't belabor all the other health issues related to smoking, except to say it seems a shame to develop a great relationship and sex, just to have your life shortened and miss ten or more years of a great life potential. For those of you who need to quit there is a program, **Quit Smoking Now!™** at the back of this book.

A clean body is a loveable body. Bathe or shower alone or together to get off the day's dirt and tensions before getting off yourselves. The smell of soap on a freshly bathed body is much more pleasant than a days worth of body odor. And if you're into oral sex it goes without saying, your partner will probably prefer a freshly washed target.

PHYSICAL AND HEALTH MATTERS...

Exercise will improve your sex

While you're at improving yourselves, there's no harm in getting into better shape. Exercise improves sex and all relationships. A healthy partner is far better than a weak, easily tiring, fragile, sickly, worn out partner. Good physical conditioning will only make you a more vigorous, active and fun person to be with. That's not just for your sexual relationship, but with your relationships with your kids, friends, fellow employees… with any and everyone. And you'll like yourself a lot better, too! If you've been a couch potato for some time, make sure you get clearance from your physician before you get into a very vigorous exercise program. Exercise as a couple and strengthen that part of your relationship too.

Medications and diseases can affect sexual activity.

There are a number of diseases and medications which can affect your sexual performance and pleasure. Among them are diabetes, hypertension, hypotension, hyperthyroidism, hypothyroidism, depression, anxiety, various circulatory disorders, cardiac problems, neurological disorders just to mention a few physical disorders. In addition, many medications diminish sexual prowess and pleasure. Among these are Bata blockers, anti-hypertensives, tranquilizers, anti-depressants, anti-seizure medications, some cold medications, sleeping pills and numerous other classes of medications. The good news is that many of these disease and medication problems can be remedied with the help of your private physician by treating the underlying cause or by adjusting medication dosage or type. ***By no means, do you stop taking your medications on your own.*** Also excessive alcohol ingestion, smoking and illicit drugs will severely reduce sexual performance, especially the ability to obtain and maintain erection.

ADVANTAGES OF SLIMMING DOWN...

Endurance

Like any activity, it is easier to move a lighter body through its paces than a weighty one. Sex can endure longer if you have to move less weight. You can move easier, faster, more agile and you'll be a lighter load for your partner to support.

A better fit

The greatest advantage of lighter, slimmer and trimmer partners is the more interesting, exciting and variety of positions you can partake in.

Tricks of the trade

Following is the real meat of this chapter … how to be the best possible lover to your partner. The following focuses on how you can give your lover the greatest possible pleasure.

Give yourself time

Quickies have their place and when the spirit moves one or both of you in a limited window of time, go for it and relieve those tensions. But too many couples seem to have nothing but quickies in their lives. Sex is important enough to your relationship that you need to give yourselves time to really express your love for each other and immerse your selves in each other's pleasure. We don't seem to have a problem setting aside adequate time for less important things than our sexual relations and what strengthens our love for each other. How much time do we waste on some ridicules sitcoms on TV, unimportant arguments, worries about things that never happen? Give yourselves an hour or more for making love from time to time and see if it isn't time better spent than most of the other things you go to the trouble of scheduling or wasting precious time at. Sure quickies have their place, but they don't hold a candle to slow, sincere, heart felt love making.

Necking is still a great starter

Do you remember how exciting your first kisses were when your love was new? Remember how exciting your necking sessions were when you were kids? Well they can be every bit as exciting and erotic now as they were in "the old days." Kissing is too often left out of love making by couples. Give yourselves time to make love ... not just get off physically. Necking is still a great way to express your feelings for each other. It's a great way to get each other in the mood, and once in the mood, it will make your sex far more erotic. Kisses should still be the turn-on they were when you first started courting.

Touch and Cuddle

Infants that do not get sufficient touching and cuddling do not thrive, bond and develop to their potential. The lack of sufficient touch and cuddle in an adult relationship will prevent it from thriving, bonding, and developing to its full potential also. We're not talking just about sexual or genital touching here; we mean hand holding, a pat or squeeze in passing each other, a meaningful hug or even a knowing wink that says, "I do love you, I'm grateful to have you, I'll never let you go!" Cuddling while you watch TV or putting an arm over your partner's shoulder, or holding hands in a movie say more about your feelings for each other than all the presents you can ever exchange. A smile or that twinkle in your eye, when you, for a moment, catch each other's glance, says volumes and can be one of the greatest turn-ons you may ever get. If those moments have faded from your relationship it's time to recapture them forthwith! Get in touch with touch!

Cuddling is proven to hold many health benefits. Cuddling is similar to massage, involving and stimulating pressure receptors under the skin which start a cascade of physiological-biochemical events including reducing the stress hormone (cortisol) and increasing immune function. Cuddling produces oxytocin the so-called "love hormone."

FOREPLAY, FOREPLAY AND MORE FOREPLAY...

Return to good old petting

Remember petting? Wow! Wasn't that fun? Before we went "all the way," petting was great! Then when we went all the way petting became "foreplay" and even the word, "foreplay" turned petting into something done as just something to get through to reach the goal of "all the way." Well we hope to change your attitude and make foreplay the best part of your love making and the "all the way" the finale to each sexual encounter.

For most men, the orgasm at the end of intercourse ends the event. For most women, multiple orgasms is a given. If foreplay is a short appetizer to the finale, most women will feel short-changed. What most men don't realize, they're getting short changed too. With a little practice and a greater emphasis on the foreplay, the good old petting, not only will women be better satisfied, but men … you too can have many multiple orgasms … and both of you will be able to build up to a far more pleasurable finale! The longer you spend in foreplay the more orgasms you will be able to achieve each building erotically on the last one, until you get to the final blast off and find out what going "all the way" can really mean!

Lubricate, lubricate, lubricate

Some women find petting irritating at the beginning, if they aren't sufficiently lubricated. As we age, natural lubrication may come about more slowly and the friction of foreplay petting can become quite uncomfortable for the female partner. This can become an immediate turn-off. To prevent this we suggest artificial lubrication at the outset of your lovemaking. Not only will artificial lubrication avoid uncomfortable, painful friction, but it will greatly increase the pleasure of foreplay. The combination of natural moisture and artificial lubrication is all the better. Furthermore, fondling of the male is far more exciting for him if done with a lubricated hand. Try it, you'll love it!

There are a number of sexual lubricants, some very expensive. Some even come flavored. Expensive doesn't make them one bit better. Flavor might cause irritation to someone with sensitivities or allergies. Our only suggestion is to avoid silicone based lubricants and use only water based products. The silicone based lubricants have a tendency to destroy some sex toys, dildos and vibrators which can be a great asset to love play. They may also cause deterioration of condoms if you use them. We'll have more to say about toys later. For now, the least expensive water based lubricants are our recommendation. You should be able to find several good brands in the $3 to $6 range.

Erotic massage

You don't have to concentrate on the genitals. A foot

massage, a shoulder or back rub can go a long way to relax your partner and help put him or her more in the mood for love and sex. Might even get rid of that "bedtime headache." Body oils can be an added pleasure, but avoid getting them into the mucosal tissues of the female genital area. Body and massage oils should not be used as vaginal lubricants.

Finger play

Fingers and hands are probably the most effective stimulators we have at our disposal. The trick is to use them in a way your partner wants most, and that can differ greatly from person to person. Some like a very gentle touch; others turn on more with a heavier touch. Some like it all. It's up to you to figure out which you partner wants. If he or she is reluctant to tell you, it's up to you to read his or her body language. If you're doing something your partner dislikes, the message should be pretty clear; lack of a pleasurable response should be a pretty clear message. On the other hand, a pleasurable response should encourage more of the same. Partners should feel free to express what's unpleasant and ask for more of what's good or great. Trial and error is the way we learn about each other and what are each other's special turn-ons.

Ladies first

Many women, perhaps all women, are one complete erogenous zone from head to toes. Lips, ears, neck, shoulders, the feet, thighs, especially the inner sides of the thighs, breasts, buttocks, tummies, all can be warm to hot zones. You needn't start right at home plate to score a run. Give yourself time to tease and please and work your way to the genital area. But let her determine how fast or slowly you get to her most erotic spots. If she shows you some impatience move on a little faster; otherwise advance as slowly as seems to give her pleasure and joy. Kisses and sincere whispers of adoration can only help.

Some women can actually achieve orgasm with stimulation of the above mentioned erogenous areas, but for most it is just a mood setter. For most women, stimulation of the genital area will finally lead her to orgasm, and for most multiple orgasms. These more intensely erotic spots include the pubic mound, the labia, clitoris, the magic G-spot, the anal area and entrance and deeper areas of the vagina.

The goal of foreplay massage to women is to give maximum pleasure to your partner and since multiple-orgasm is a more normal achievement for women there is really no reason to avoid her orgasms during foreplay. When foreplay orgasms do occur they are usually more expanded, more intense and more satisfying as they continue.

Gently massage the legs, abdomen, thighs, breasts, any and all her special erogenous areas other than her genitals, to encourage her to relax. Use adequate lubricant on her pubic mound and pelvic area. Begin gently massaging the mound and outer lips of the *genital area.* Spend time and do not rush. Relax and enjoy her gradually increasing pleasure responses and giving the massage. Gently squeeze the outer lip between your fingers, sliding up and down the entire length of each of her lips. Do the same to her inner vaginal lips of her vagina. Take your time and don't forget kisses if they help excite her. She should feel comfortable telling you what pleasures her most; speed, depth, the pressure needed to be increased or decreased.

The clitoris is similar to the male's glans penis (head of the penis) but is over four times more sensitive. Its tip portion holds up to 8,000 sensory nerve endings, more than any other area of the body. This wonderfully sensitive spot has only one purpose; for sheer pleasure! Stroking the clitoris with clockwise and counter-clockwise circles as well as lengthwise and with varying pressures will give extreme pleasure, but because of its sensitivity adequate lubrication is essential. *Lack of enough lubrication will quickly turn pleasure to irritation.* Gently squeeze it between thumb and index fingers. If she orgasms, great ... she'll probably have many more to come!

Slowly insert a finger into the vagina. Slowly and gently massage the inside of the vagina. Move slowly, gently, up, down, sideways, around the entrance, then deeper. Lubricate adequately. Move your finger in a "come here" gesture. You will feel a spongy area of tissue just behind the pubic bone, above the clitoris. This is her G-spot. In reality it is more a G area and it will actually engorge when stimulated enlarging to as much as a square inch or more. She may feel the need to urinate, but hopefully she'll only feel sheer pleasure. Vary the pressure, speed and pattern of movement; move side to side, back and forth, or in circles with your finger. Be even more pleasurable for her, but if this causes an uncomfortable stretch for her, back off. Most women should have no problem and might enjoy the increased stimulation from two or more fingers. Take your time; be very gentle. Use your thumb to stimulate the clitoris as well. If she has an orgasm, let her recover briefly, then continue massaging if she wants. More orgasms should occur, each gaining in intensity. And her ecstasy should turn you on more than any little pill can!

Let's not forget the man

Ladies, your man's erection and pleasure is your responsibility. Just as it is his responsibility to get you turned on, so is his pleasure and ability to perform your responsibility. A great deal of his excitement and erection will probably come in response to your reaction to his pleasuring you, but fondling and caressing him will certainly heighten his pleasure and reaction. Kisses, hugs, holding him close to you, rubbing against him and sincere words of endearment and praise are bound to add inches and vigor to his member. Lips, ears, neck, shoulders, back, feet, inner thighs and buttocks are erogenous zones as well for men, but usually not as sensitive as for women.

For him, getting right to the point will usually do fine, but if he has some special pleasure spots do your best to find them and use them to your advantage. As mentioned before, stimulation of his penis with lubricant in your hand will heighten his pleasure. Furthermore, the penis has more sensitive areas for pleasuring him. Most sensitive is the end or head of the penis. Also the underside of the shaft is usually highly sensitive. These are areas to concentrate on if he needs more effort to get hard and fully erect and areas to ease off on if you sense he is getting too close to orgasm. It is this control which you will later learn to help him avoid premature ejaculation as well as achieving multiple orgasms. You have a heavy responsibility!

The goal of penis massage in this situation is not to achieve orgasm, but to give foreplay pleasure, create erection and prepare for intercourse. This foreplay should also including fondling of the testicles, (carefully please), perineum and externally the prostate. If the man has a problem with performance anxiety this foreplay should help relax him and eventually reduce such fears. On the occasional times when the male partner needs sexual gratification when his partner is incapacitated or just not in the mood, this massage will certainly get the job done and let him achieve a most pleasurable orgasm, or two, or three, or more.

You may want to start by gently massaging his shoulders, back, legs, abdomen, thighs, chest, nipples, to get the receiver to relax and tease him a bit. Use lubricant on the shaft and head of his penis and testicles, gently massaging the testicles, making sure not to cause pressure and pain. Massage the pubic area above the penis. Massage the perineum, the area between the testicles and anus as this gives pressure on the prostate. Slowly massaging the shaft of the penis, vary your speed and pressure. Gently squeeze the penis at the base with your hand, pull up and slide off, then alternate with your other hand. Repeat this frequently. For a change of pace, change the direction starting the squeeze at the head or glans penis sliding down and off, alternating hands. You should get great pleasure watching his pleasure and response. It's not unusual for a partner to start this stimulation because of not being in the mood and upon watching his arousal and pleasure getting turned on, leading to mutual sex play or intercourse.

Massage the head of the penis gently as this area has the most nerve endings and may be very sensitive. Remember, the purpose of this massage is probably not to reach a wet orgasm, but to prepare for eventual intercourse. Use sufficient lubricant. If excitement gets too great and you suspect he is approaching a final or wet orgasm, ease off and let him relax and cool down, have a dry orgasm. When your partner has eased off, start again by massaging all around the head and penis shaft. The penis may or may not soften as you ease off to let him cool down. It may get soft then hard, then soft and hard again, several times which is a highly desirable

If you feel he is going to ejaculate, back off, allowing his penis to soften a little before resuming the massage. Repeat this several times, coming close to ejaculation, and then backing off. This will eventually lead to the ability to achieve multiple orgasms for him.

More about that later! Remember the goal is not orgasm but to prolong his pleasure and prepare for intercourse. More importantly, this will help him to learn control of orgasm and to become multi-orgasmic. By learning the art of ejaculatory control, coming close to ejaculation and then backing off, he will become multi-orgasmic. There is a small area midway between the testicles and anus. You can massage his penis with one hand and massage this spot with the other. Pressing on this spot when he nears ejaculation will help him ease off of wet orgasm.

Premature Ejaculation

There is little agreement about the definition or cause of premature ejaculation, and no one really understands how the treatments work. But be that as it may treatment of premature ejaculation is 95% to 98% percent effective. Of all the sexual dysfunction, one can acquire, this is the best to have.

The Psychiatric Association defines premature ejaculation as *"ejaculation with minimal sexual stimulation or before, upon, or shortly after penetration and before the person wishes it."* However, a couple who engages in 45 minutes of unrestrained manual and oral-genital foreplay, followed by one minute of pleasurable intercourse, would not be considered by us to be cursed by premature ejaculation. Premature ejaculation is typically a younger man's problem, the majority of cases involving men under the age of 30. Premature ejaculation is common in young men in their first sexual experiences and might be considered perfectly normal. With increased sexual experience, most men get over their initial premature ejaculation spontaneously.

Whatever the definition or cause of premature ejaculation might be, the treatment is quite effective. The *"pause"* and the *"squeeze"* procedures developed by Masters and Johnson, are highly effective. Success rates of 90 to 98 percent can be realistically expected. In the *pause* procedure, the penis should be manually stimulated to fairly high arousal. The couple then pauses until his arousal subsides, then stimulation is resumed. This is repeated often as possible before stimulation is carried on to ejaculation. Thus the man experiences much more total time of stimulation before ejaculation. The squeeze, like the stop-start, requires intermission of stimulation, adding that as stimulation stops, the partner firmly squeezes the penis between her thumb and forefinger, below where the head of the penis joins the shaft further reducing arousal. Following a few weeks of this the man is able to experience more continuous penile stimulation without ejaculating.

Next, the couple progresses to penetrating the penis into the vagina but without intense thrusting movements. If the man rapidly becomes highly aroused, the penis is withdrawn. The couple waits for arousal to subside, and penis is reinserted. When good tolerance for inactive containment of the penis is achieved, the procedure is repeated with active thrusting.

Drugs and medications that block the sympathetic nervous system may have the effect of delaying ejaculation. These include anti-anxiety, antidepressant, and major tranquilizing medications; sedatives; some medications used to treat high blood pressure; and some antihistamines. Because of serious side effects, the use of medication in treating premature ejaculation is not recommended, especially when the effectiveness of the behavioral retraining procedure is usually so successful. .

SLICKY LICKY...

Cunnilingus

This is oral sex on a woman. The partner stimulates the genital area with lips and tongue is usually very highly erotic, stimulating and exciting to most women and to some, the quickest rout to orgasm. However, oral sex is also very individual; to some women it is unpleasant, offensive and even repulsive. It should never be forced. If your partner is opposed to this form of sexual expression, talk about it. Many women are quite concerned about feminine odor or body image. It may be a matter of fearing you will find her unclean or with offensive odor or she may be sensitive about the appearance of her genital area. Bathing or showering should eliminate this problem, but many women do not realize that the normal genital taste and fragrance is very erotic to the male. It is the stimulant to sexual action in the animal kingdom and we are part of that kingdom.

It may be that she feels you will expect her to return the favor of oral sex and this may worry her. The thought of ejaculating into her mouth can be a turn-off. If she can have confidence that you will stop before ejaculating, it may solve that problem. Also the use of a condom for Fellatio to catch the emission may be helpful. In any case, open communication is essential in this matter as it is in all sexual practices.

Fellatio

This is the fancy name of oral sex on a man. There is little resistance for this activity by men. However, as mentioned above, there might be resistance by his partner. Again, good hygienic habits can go a long way toward helping resolve this resistance. Also earning her confidence that you will not ejaculate into her mouth, if this offends her, will be helpful. Communication of fears or feelings about oral sex is important in understanding each other's feelings about any sexual activities.

High tech electronics… toys, toys. Toys

Vibrators, dildos and all forms of sex toys have never been more available than today and their wide spread use, especially by women, both single and married, has made them an extremely profitable product. "Sex toy parties" have started to replace the Tupper Ware parties. Sex toy showers are replacing kitchen showers for the brides to be. These items have been popular among single women for some time, but they are becoming an important and fun part of foreplay among couples. They are extremely stimulating, and are helpful in making women with difficult orgasm turn into multi-orgasmic beings. There are vibrating "cock rings" to help men with some difficulty achieving erection to harden and maintain erection.

Vibrators are not a new invention. They were originally developed in the late 1800's as a medical device that doctors used to treat hysteria in women. The accepted treatment for this problem then was to bring on orgasm. Vibrators were invented so that doctors or their nurses could more easily and quickly treat these women! It's a fact, *Believe It Or Not!*

Some women have complained that their partners have

shown jealousy and have gotten upset by their use of these helpful devices. In most cases, such feelings are defused when the toys are used together as part of foreplay, the partner administrating the pleasure to his mate and seeing what joy and satisfaction the loved one achieves. As with any sexual activity, lubricate, lubricate, lubricate. For those interested, there are numerous stores specializing in the sale of these devices, or if you prefer shopping in private and desire plain unmarked wrappers, the internet has an abundance of merchants, and often their prices are considerably better. Shop around for the lowest prices and get a titillating education at the same time.

Anal action

Like oral sex, anal sex is a very individual activity. It is a sexual practice which is fine if it is consensual. It must never be forced and if it causes physical or mental pain for either partner it should be avoided until and if such difficulties can be resolved.

There are several degrees of anal action, from mere fondling, to digital penetration, licking, sex-toy penetration to actual penetration with the penis. If anal action is an activity you wish to try as a couple, start with simple fondling and advance slowly by degree until both of you are comfortable in its exploration. Most important is that you practice extreme hygiene, emptying the bowel and cleansing the anal area carefully. Lubricate, lubricate, lubricate.... Do not use sharp objects or toys that could perforate the sensitive rectal tissues. Always use condoms. Never penetrate the vagina with any toy, or appendage that has not been thoroughly cleaned after being in the anus.

Sex after 50 … It's never ever too late

Survey of married men and women showed that 87% of married men and 89% of married women in the 60-64 age range are sexually active. Those numbers drop with advancing years, but 29% of men and 25% of women over the age of 80 are still sexually active. These figures would probably be higher if one or the other partner weren't hindered by infirmities or if opportunity presented to widows or widowers. Older age can be a time of freedom to explore sexual expression in ways never before possible. And it seems to be very healthy too. Recent studies showed that men who have more than two orgasms per week have lower mortality statistics.

There are numerous ways in which men and women can adapt to aging changes and continue to be, or become, a sexually active. Realize that sexual arousal takes longer and requires more manual stimulation. Take all the time that you often didn't have in younger years to pleasure each other or yourself. Share what makes you feel good with your partner. Take time to explore all the tactile, visual, auditory, and even olfactory aspects of intimacy. Make adequate lubrication part of your routine, to avoid irritation of the vagina or painful intercourse. A water-based lubricant is best; oil-based lubricants and petroleum products such as Vaseline may be difficult to flush out of the vagina, possibly causing irritation or infection. You should make applying the lubricant part of your lovemaking routine. If the above suggestions are not sufficient to help you achieve the level of activity you desire, ask for help; your primary care doctor, urologist, or gynecologist may be able to help, or may refer you to a sex therapist or a sex coach.

Some men and women may question whether age can affect the chances of success in becoming multi-orgasmic. There is no reason sexually mature men or women of any age shouldn't find success, as long as they are capable of being sexually active. If you have no trouble reaching orgasms, either with a partner or by yourself, then becoming multi-orgasmic should only be a matter of patience, determination, and practice. In fact, studies have shown that women often become more orgasmic as they age up and through their ninth decade.

MULTIPLE ORGASMS

Female

Dry orgasms are almost a given for women in this past decade. For most women in their mature years multiple orgasms is probably the norm. Certainly to be non-orgasmic should not be considered the norm for any woman and should be addressed. No woman should have to miss this important fulfilling pleasure.

Yes, males too can have Multiple Dry Orgasms

With a basic understanding of male sexuality and practice of some simple techniques virtually any man can become multi-orgasmic. First step is to change the focus of sex from the goal of ejaculating, to that of love making. Once becoming multi-orgasmic, the male will not only enjoy sex far more himself, but also will much more satisfy and gratify his partner.

Male multiple orgasms will occur in succession, without loss of sexual arousal between each. Fortunately, women are usually blessed with the ability to have multiple orgasms effortlessly. Men can actually achieve the same blessing. The multi-orgasmic male does not completely lose his erection or desire between orgasms. *Orgasm and ejaculation are actually two separate happenings.* Ejaculation is actually the emission of seminal fluid <u>after </u>orgasm. *Multiple male orgasms are orgasms without ejaculation until the end of very last orgasm of the specific sexual experience.*

It will be helpful to understand the process of male sexual arousal cycle as first described by **Masters & Johnson.**

The Excitement Phase

1.Vaso-congestion and erection of the penis; the flow of blood into the penis at a higher rate than the outflow causing erection.
2. Increased heart rate
3. Tumescence; the partial elevation of the testacies and increase in their size
4. Nipple erection

The Plateau Phase

1. Further increase in penis and testicle size
2. Further testicular elevation
3. Purple hue and swelling of the glans (tip or head) of the penis
4. Cowper's gland secretions; a male natural lubricant
5. Hyperventilation

The Orgasm Phase

Pre-ejaculation phase; sperm and fluid are expelled from the vas deferens, seminal vesicles and prostate gland, causing seminal fluid to collect at the base of the urethral bulb near the prostate.
1. Myotonia - muscular rigidity, further swelling and lengthening of the penis just before the release tension
2. Blood pressure and respiratory rate increase further.

Ejaculation - the point of no return

1. Bladder sphincter closes tightly to prevent seminal backflow into the bladder
2. Rhythmic contractions of the prostate, perennial muscles and penile shaft propel semen outward as the ejaculate

Resolution Phase

1. Reversal in myotonia and vasocongestion
2. Erection loss
3. Relaxation of the scrotum and testes descend
4. Reduction of heart rate and lowering blood pressure.

> **It is important to realize that orgasm and ejaculation are two very separate and distinct events.**

Multiple orgasms as apposed to ejaculatory orgasms

Both types of orgasm begin in the same way, from arousal to a point near ejaculation, the *"point of no return"*. At this point, a man will experience a series of genital contractions lasting three to five seconds, known as pelvic orgasms. This *pelvic orgasm* feels like a fluttering or mild release of pressure. Identifying and controlling, these sensations is the key to male multiple orgasm. Each multiple orgasm will become progressively more intense and pleasurable until the final ejaculatory orgasm which you will allow when you and your partner are ready for the finale.

These pre-ejaculatory orgasms are also known as dry orgasms, even though there may be a small amount of leakage of seminal fluid with some of them. The key to controlling and achieving multiple dry orgasms is when you are approaching *your* point of no return, is not to *spill* over into an ejaculation but to decrease stimulation long enough to gain control back to the arousal stage. This control is achieved by squeezing the *pubococcygeal* muscle or pelvic floor muscles. These are the same muscles you contract when stopping urinating in mid-stream.

The *plateau stage* is the heightened state of arousal which will eventually lead into pre-ejaculatory dry orgasm and ejaculatory *orgasm* if stimulation is allowed to continue. Once the plateau phase is reached, it is passed rather quickly as the orgasm builds and ejaculation occurs. In a multiple orgasmic encounter, the plateau phase is reached and allowed to enter into a dry orgasm. The dry orgasm is pleasurable but does not completely discharge the sexual energy and arousal and lose the penile erection though there will be some reduction of tension and stiffness momentarily. There will be a short refractory period, from a few seconds to a minute or two and then the plateau stage will start to build again to another dry orgasm. The successive dry orgasms will be slightly stronger than the previous ones. Once you have mastered control over your orgasms, you will be able to continue multiple dry orgasms until you and your partner decide it time to ejaculate in a finale orgasm.

Achieving male dry multiple orgasms

They are so closely related that most men have thought them one and the same. In fact, ejaculation is the event that occurs at the end of orgasm. It is the climax after orgasm that ends the man's ability to continue effective sexual activity. It is what turns a dry orgasm into a final wet orgasm. The first and most important step is for you to learn to distinguish between the two.

The ability to separate these events involves the *pubococcygeal* muscle, or pelvic floor muscle. This is the muscle you use to stop the flow of urine in mid-stream. This muscle can be strengthened by repeated flexion of the muscle as you would with repeated interruption of urination. It will feel as if your entire pelvis and its contents are being drawn up. It's essential to become familiar with this muscle and learn to control it at will. Control will come with experience and by strengthening it through regular exercise.

Practice makes perfect

This can be done with your partner's fondling and manipulation or on your own through masturbation. Remember that orgasm and ejaculation are two very distinct and separate events. You can learn to distinguish and separate these two phases though the transition from one to the other is short. It is because they occur in such rapid succession that most men have accepted orgasm and ejaculation as one

1. Begin love making with your partner or masturbating as you would normally building to the *plateau stage*. You and your partner should learn to identify this stage by body language, the change in your height of your excitement, the further hardening and swelling of your penis and you telling her to stop stimulation.

2. Stop just before reaching your point of no return that point at which you would otherwise ejaculate. At this point contract and hold your pelvic floor muscle until your immediate excitement level eases. Allow yourself relax and take a several moments break.

3. When you are a bit more relaxed, but before you lose your erection, begin again, this time trying to bringing you just a bit closer to the point of no return, and again contracting your pelvic muscle to prevent ejaculation.
4. Continue this cycle of arousal and interruption paying very special attention to your state of emotional feelings and arousal. The more you and your partner learn about your sexual response the sooner you'll be in control your orgasmic response.

Don't be discouraged if at first you miss the signals to stop stimulation and accidentally have a wet orgasm. Take advantage of this by you and your partner trying to notice the subtle changes which take place just before ejaculation takes place. Even as you start to ejaculate, squeeze your pelvic muscles and try to stop the wet orgasm. You may be able to shorten the ejaculation and reduce the refractory period. Remember, this practice is fun, even if at first it fails. More practice is more fun and makes perfect. With continued practice, you will learn the necessary timing and control.

Once in control of your dry orgasms you should be able to suppress ejaculation until your partner is completely satisfied, regardless of how long she needs pleasuring and satisfying; hours if necessary.

> Don't let anyone tell you that sex is no longer a need for someone your age!

Rekindling the flames

Make terrific lemonade out of what you thought was a lemon. It may take a little longer but that's a terrific advantage.

Many elderly couples will tell you sex has never been better. Women, especially appreciate the fact that their partners are slower to orgasm and can keep up with them longer to satisfy them more completely. More foreplay, more orgasms seem to become the rule for successful sexual relationships. Relationships, like good wine, seem to mellow and get better with age. A new closeness seems to bloom with time.

How often is not enough … too much … just right?

Frequency of sex is as individual as any other aspect of a healthy sexual relationship. There is no correct number; if you are both satisfied with once a month then once a month is just fine, if twice or more a day is fine with both of you that's fine too. It's when one wants it twice a day and one wants it once a month that you may have a conflict. Compromise will probably be required. If your differences are really that great, counseling will possibly be needed. Chances are that differences will not be so extreme that a couple will be able to work things out themselves. The important thing is to recognize that there is no necessarily right sexual frequency. If each partner feels free to be the aggressor when the mood dictates, then that will probably help you to find your ideal frequency.

Othniel Seiden, MD & Jane L. Bilett, Ph.D.

WIDOWERS, WIDOWS,
SINGLES AND SAFE SEX

Meeting a new partner

If you've been out of circulation for a long time, having been with one partner for a prolonged time, getting back into circulation can be difficult as well as scary. You've probably been comfortably confident with your long time partner but starting new relationships can have lots of self-searching questions. How will I respond to a new partner? How will a new partner respond to me? How will I know we will be mutually right for each other? How can I meet someone who will be right for me? There are lots of sources of advice out there, as much poor as good: Church, synagogue, mosque, health clubs, bars, dance studios, adult education classes, the grocery store, the internet, fix-ups by friends, relatives and co-workers, etc., etc., etc. Which are best, which should I steer clear of?

Bars are probably the least safe place to find a trusting partner that you want to spend your future with. Probably the best idea is to let your own interests lead you to partner you'll get on with well. If your religion is a top priority your church, synagogue or mosque may be the place to start your search. If you are a health fanatic, head for the health club. Adult education classes of interest to you may also interest the right partner for you.

Special mention should be made of the internet dating services. They are usually good at limiting matches as to age, interests, religions, intentions such as dating, long term relationships, matrimony, etc., BUT they are only as good as the honesty of the person replying to your query. Believe it or not, some married men have been known to sign on to these services as singles, and almost as unbelievable, some responders have lied about their ages. Unbelievable!

Occasionally someone might even place a photo of themselves that is twenty years old. However, these are the exception rather than the rule. To make things safer for participants, only e-mail addresses are usually required and e-mail correspondence can be used to get to know each other a little better. If is decided to finally meet it is wise to meet at a public place for coffee, a meal or a safe location for a face-to-face chat. We utilized the internet. Otti had been widowed for about a year. Jane tried it after 8 years being divorced. Otti had about half-a-dozen coffee dates and Jane was number seven. We eventually married. The internet obviously worked for us.

Safe sex

Deciding to become sexually intimate with a partner can be a big step to take in any relationship, especially since, for many people, having sex involves an emotional commitment as well as a physical one.

If you have been recently widowed or divorced from a long marriage, you must consider a serious change that has taken place possibly since you last took a partner. HIV may not have been around when you last dated someone other than your past spouse. The decision to become sexually intimate with a new partner must also be considered with HIV and other sexually transmitted diseases (STDs) now more prevalent among our population. Too often infections are asymptomatic, so transmitting the disease to another person may occur unknowingly. Other than abstinence, only a barrier method, like condoms or dental dams in the case of oral sex, can reduce transmission of HIV and certain other STDs among non-monogamous partners. Abstinence is the only completely effective method of preventing STDs, HIV and pregnancy.

A sobering statistic points out that the *fastest growing*

population now being diagnosed with HIV and new STDs is the over 60 age group!

Complete monogamy is the only way to feel secure regarding transmission of diseases. In the case of HIV, even a blood test is not assurance until partners have been monogamous for over six to eight months. Engaging in sexual intercourse with a relative stranger can be scary or dangerous in this day and age; discussing both the emotional and physical risks of sex and deciding with your new partner how best to minimize those risks can be can make for an even more intimate sexual experience.

Practicing safe sex doesn't mean eliminating sex from your life. What practicing safe sex means is showing consideration, love, concern, and respect for partners and for you. Safer sex means enjoying sex to the fullest without transmitting, or acquiring, sexually related infections. There are numerous sexually transmissible diseases; but the consequences of HIV and syphilis, may be deadly. All STD's are caused by microorganisms which pass between partners during particular sexual activities.

CHAPTER 15

INVOLVE OTHERS...

The surest way to keep you on the proper course is to lead others on the same quest. Certainly you want the longest, healthiest, happiest life for your family and loved ones. Well, what's good for you is good for them. Your spouse should be accompanying you on your pursuit. So should your children. It's never too early to begin a healthy lifestyle. And it is rarely ever too late to turn over a new leaf. Your parents, and if you're lucky enough to still have grandparents, they should all start working to retain what good health they have, correct what ailments they are afflicted with and do all they can to prevent premature deterioration.

Another way to involve others is to start a support group at your job, at your health club, YMCA, church, synagogue, or among your neighbors and friends. Not only will it keep you focused on your goal, it will win you many new friends. Gather to work out together on a regular schedule and ride herd on each other's progress. Help each other over the tough times when for one reason or another someone slips off the wagon. You'll fine that "the more the merrier" is the truth.

Put the word out with a simple flyer or place an announcement in your church or office newsletter. If there's a neighborhood weekly or advertiser, a blurb in it will get you lots of participants. The expense shouldn't be too great, and they may publish it free for you as a public service. **Start a senior citizen's version of "Our Gang!"**

CHAPTER 16

ECONOMICS OF AGE....

When Social Security was introduced over half a century ago, no one expected you and 75,000 or more of you to live a full century. You were supposed to start getting paid your pension at 65 and die at 68 or there about. Well I'm not about to co-operate with the government's idea of "Golden Years." If you fall anywhere near the average, you'll get somewhere around $500 to $600 a month, around $1,000 to $1200 per couple if you retire at 62 years of age. To supplement that, you'll be able to earn around $8,000 to $9,000 a year, after which you'll have to pay back $1 for every $2 you earn over your limit. Retire at 65 and they'll pay you back at a rate of $600 to $1700 per month and you'll be able to earn a little more before they start taking it back.

At the age 70, you'll be able to earn all you want without payback—if they don't change the rules by then. (*Guess what? They've changed it!*) In any case, life on Social Security ain't gonna be easy!

So what can you do about it?

Hopefully you have some savings, a Keogh Plan, a 401K, a pension from work, stocks, bonds, a home with paid up mortgage—some kind of nest egg squirreled away, a tin can full of $1000 bills buried in the back yard! If yes or no, let's look at the options.

Actuarial tables of insurance companies even say that a

man retiring at age 65 can look forward to at least 15 years of retirement and women at the same age over twenty years. These are conservative estimates. With the lifestyle changes people are making today, with the advances in medical care and growth in other technologies, the 65 year old who exercises, follows sensible nutrition, doesn't smoke and poison his or her system with other chemical abuses should far exceed those predictions. Don't forget, those actuarial tables are made up of averages of those who make wise lifestyle choices and those who make bad choices. For those who make the bad choices and die below the ages of 80 and 85 there are those who balance the average and far outlive those actuarial ages. Because you are reading this book, you are making the wise choices. It would also be wise to plan for a life span of 50 more years—or greater!

So how much money will you need to carry you through life in the style to which you're accustomed? A rule of the thumb which pops up in most books on retirement states that on the average, "The cost of living during retirement is about 70% to 80% of what you needed before retirement. Why so much less? Most retirees no longer have to put kids through school, they have their home paid off, they carry less insurance, they need less new clothing, they can get by on one car, they entertain less, make fewer major purchases, don't have as many loans with high interest rates, etc., etc., etc. Again these are averages and some will do better, others will exceed these expenditures.

So how do we prepare?

Take inventory!

Study!

Get good advice!

Consider later retirement or partial retirement!

Retrain and retrench!

Take inventory....

What are your assets? Inquire of the Social Security Administration for an estimate of your social security payments when you and your spouse retire at certain ages, 62, 65, or 70. It could vary between $500 to $1800 a month for each of you depending on how long you worked and how much you contributed during those years.

Estimate what you will get from pensions from employers, IRAs, 401Ks, savings, investments, royalties, etc.

Add to these estimates the value of your home equity. The sum of these figures will be roughly what you will have to rely on to retire. How long will it carry you? How can you stretch it? What can you do to supplement it? These are the next questions you have to ask yourself. Don't panic quite yet! It may not be as bad as it seems.

Study....

Your local library probably has dozens of books on financing your retirement. Check them all out and study them. Lots of them will tell you how to retire well if you're a millionaire, some will address the problems facing those of us who didn't make it to even a quarter of that wealth. They will show you how to figure your true net worth and it may surprise you that you are better off than you think. Further more, if you are now around fifty, they will suggest how to prepare yourself in the next twelve to twenty years to get the maximum nest egg for retirement. If you've read this book to here and follow its preaching, make it 40 to 50 years.

Get good advice....

There are lots of financial advisors out there waiting and willing to give you advice on how to maximize your future fortune. Some are good at what they do, too many are totally unqualified. Get referrals from people who have had good success with their financial advisors. Shy away from an advisor who benefits from commissions by buying and selling your stocks and bonds. Ask your accountant for advice and referrals. Listen to the advice, then weigh it and think about it before you jump. Discuss it with others whose opinions you respect. Most advice is cheap and only worth its weight in dust, good advise is worth its weight in gold.

Consider later retirement or partial retirement....

If you like the work you're doing and are healthy, seriously consider delaying your retirement. You have lots of years between now and the end of your century for golf, fishing and travel. Every extra year you work, you can enlarge that nest egg rather than draw on it. And remember, if you take retirement at 70 instead of 62 or 65, your social security payment grows—if they don't change the rules. You have to consider that possibility

If you don't like the job you have or don't want to put in all the hours you now do, consider partial retirement. Look at a new job with less pressure and hours. Use your newfound time and available space to create *passive income* streams. Perhaps something you've always wanted to try but couldn't afford to take the pay cut. Now may be the chance you've waited for. Less pressure, less pay, more free time, doing something new you've always wanted to do, yet still building or at least supplementing the nest egg. It's worth considering and discussing with your financial advisor.

Retrain and retrench....

If you take social security and don't want to earn over your allotted limit you may want to consider retraining or developing new skills for the time when you will again be allowed to earn more. Perhaps real estate school, training for stock broker's license or some other job which interests you and lets you pick and choose your hours and your earning potential. Think about teaching. Take a hard look at volunteer work. It won't put money in your pocket, but it will give you great satisfaction and can often lead to part time paid work either through the organization you are volunteering for or through the connections you make.

Retirement does not mean itinerant....

In the past, retirement raised the image of an old fogy rocking in a chair watching as the world goes by—or nowadays more likely watching TV soaps and sitcoms. That's not what your next thirty to fifty years should be all about. Retirement should be a whole new opportunity, not a dead end. It's as much a time to start a new career, pursue hobbies which can turn into careers, travel get more active than you've ever been before. The worst thing you can do is just sit there and watch your savings dwindle.

You've spent probably half a century getting to where you are today. In that time you've learned a lot. Now use that hard earned knowledge to make the **second half which starts a fifty** an active, productive, **happy golden time of life!**

ABOUT THE AUTHOR(S)

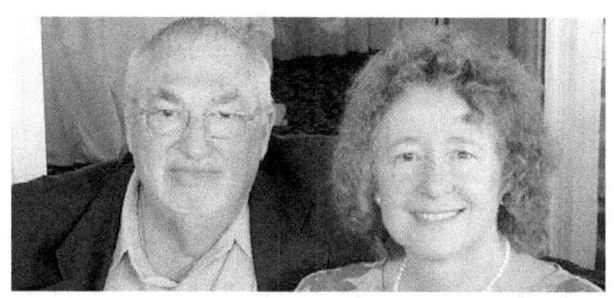

OTHNIEL J. SEIDEN, M.D.
JANE L. BILETT, PH.D.

As one of the medical professionals in the charitable organization "Doctors To The World," Othniel Seiden has seen many cultures and made many amazing discoveries. His fascination about the longevity of the population in third world countries was of particular interest. He was uniquely positioned to study the phenomenon people who the West would typically classify as poor living to 100 and even 120.

He studied their diets, their lifestyle and their beliefs and began to understand what factors help them to achieve such long lives. As a physician, Othniel colors those findings and applies them to the lifestyles of the Western world.

Weaving in Jane Bilett's psychotherapy research, these two authors show us not only why it is possible to achieve a life span of 120, but that it can be achieved by some simple lifestyle changes.

More From Othniel

Health

5 HTP The Serotonin Connection:
*The Natural Supplement that helps
you be in control of your mind and body!*
ISBN: 1519148445

5-HTP and Depression Management:
Available in Kindle Only

5HTP and Memory Loss Management with:
Available in Kindle Only

5 HTP PMS and Menopause:
Available in Kindle Only

Coping with Arthritis:
ISBN: 151941353X

Coping with BPH:
*Benign Prostatic Hypertrophy
Male, over 45, you probably have it!*
Available in Kindle Only

Coping with Colorectal Cancer:
*Prevention and Cure of theSecond Leading
Cause of Cancer Deaths*
Available in Kindle Only

Coping with Fibromyalgia:
It's not in your head, it's a disease!
ISBN: 1519438311

Coping with Prostate Cancer:
*Prevention and Cure
of Man's Most Common Cancer*
ISBN: 1519438737

Heart of a Woman:
>*Prevetion and Cure of the #1 Killer in Women*
>>**ISBN: 1519441533**

Heavy and Healthy:
>*Forget Your Weight and Get Fit!*
>>**ISBN: 1519495412**

Quit Smoking Now!:
>*The Program to Help You*
>*Quit Smoking Now and Forever!*
>>**ISBN: 1519495781**

Sharpening the Aging Mind:
>*Methods, Tricks & Tips to*
>*Keep Your Mind Super Sharp*
>>**ISBN: 1519496028**

Sleep Disorders Management:
>>**Available in Kindle Only**

The Second half begins at 50:
>*Your Longevity Handbook*
>>**ISBN: 1519496389**

Walk!:
>*Walk Your Way to Great Health & Long Life*
>>**Available in Kindle Only**

Weight & Appetite Management:
>>**Available in Kindle Only**

Relationships:

Adultery Case Histories:
>*Why People Cheat on Their Partners*
>>**Available in Kindle Only**

Communing with the Dead:
>*Death Needn't Part You*
>>**ISBN: 1519190085**

Foreplay:
> *The True Focus of Great Sex*
> **ISBN: 1519440979**

Sex in the Golden Years:
> *The Best Sex Ever, Stay Sexually Active for Life*
> **ISBN: 1519495927**

The Big O:
> *Male & Female Multiple Orgasms*
> **ISBN: 1519496109**

The Hospice Experience:
> *Making Your Most Important Final Decision*
> **ISBN: 1519496281**

When Your Spouse Dies:
> *A widow's & widower's handbook*
> **ISBN: 151949646X**

Jewish Fiction

Padre Pio:
> *The Capuchin – the life of Padre Pio -*
> *St. Pio of Pietrelcina*
> *Sex, Horror & Violence vs. Unyielding Faith!*
> **ISBN: 1519495684**

Seed of Avraham:
> *A 4000 Year History of the Jewish Family...*
> **ISBN: 1519495811**

Shtetl:
> *The Story of a Life No More...*
> *As told from the hereafter*
> **ISBN: 1519496036**

The Cartographer:
> *1492*
> > **ISBN: 151949615X**

The Condemned Voyage:
> *The S.S. St. Louis - 1939*
> > **Available in Kindle Only**

The Crusades:
> *The Jewish World of the 12th Century*
> > **Available in Kindle Only**

The Death of Berlin:
> *A Story of Hollocaust Survival and Revenge*
> > **Available in Kindle Only**

The Remnant:
> *The Jewish Resistance in WWII*
> > **ISBN: 1519496346**

The Uprising of Babi Yar:
> *The Syrets Deathcamp*
> > **Available in Kindle Only**

Miscellaneous

Guaranteed Routes to Success for Writers:
> *A Road Map Through Today's*
> *Dramatic Changes in Publishing*
> > **Available in Kindle Only**

Joy of Volunteering:
> *Working and Surviving in Developing Countries*
> > **ISBN: 1519495587**

So You Want to Write a Book:
> > **ISBN: 1519496079**

APPENDIX I.

YOUR PERSONAL IMPROVEMENT CHARTS.

Measure these parameters once a month and record them to follow your improvement.

Month	1	2	3	4	5	6	7	8	9	Resting Pulse
Blood Pressure										
Waist Size										
Thigh Size										
Hip Size										
Chest Size										
Neck Size										
Body Fat										

Your Walking Record:

When you first begin walking, walk as far and as long as is comfortable for you up to one hour if you can. Record the time and distance at the end of each progressive week. Then try to add to the time and the distance each day until you are able to walk briskly for an hour with confidence.

You will probably be able to walk briskly for one hour long before eight weeks have passed. As soon as you are able to walk briskly for an hour, begin taking your pulse at the middle of your walk and once more just before you begin your cool down. Take your pulse for 10 seconds and multiply it by 6. Average the two results and record it once a week. On the day you take your recording pulses, also record your time and distance for that day. Gradually increase your walking speed until you are able to maintain your Ideal Exercise Pulse Rate for your age for one hour.

As your physical condition improves you will notice that the distance you walk in one hour to maintain the same Ideal Exercise Pulse rate will lengthen. After you achieve a high level of physical fitness your improvement will slow and you may only want to record your progress once a month.

Week	1	2	3	4	5	6	7	8
Time Walked								
Distance Walked								

Week	1	2	3	4	5	6	7	8	9	10
Distance 1 Hour										
Walking Pulse Rate										

Month	1	2	3	4	5	6	7	8	9	10
Distance 1 Hour										
Walking Pulse Rate										

Month	11	12	13	14	15	16	17	18	19	20
Distance 1 Hour										
Walking Pulse Rate										

If you liked

Second Half Begins at 50

Please leave a review on
Amazon.com

Also available in Kindle